SANUM Therapy
according to Prof. Enderlein

by Günter Weigel,
Naturopath

A Comprehensive Guide

to

SANUM Therapy

according to Prof. Enderlein

---

by Günter Weigel, Naturopath

Disclaimer

The purpose of this book is to provide information about the use of SANUM preparations for a wide range of medical problems. However, illness can be highly unpredictable, and the best possible expertise should always be consulted. No liability is accepted by the author and publishers for any claims arising from the use of any remedy or prescribing strategy discussed here. remedy or prescribing strategy discussed here.

Published by Semmelweis-Verlag, D-27316 Hoya

Buchumschlag: Y. Harste
Printed in Germany by Druckerei Adam Prettenhofer GmbH & Co. KG

1st Edition 2001

Acknowledgements

I would like to express my thanks here to all who have helped me on the way to understanding the fascinating and marvellous SANUM therapy according to Prof. Enderlein:

Naturopath Franz Arnoul for introducing me to SANUM therapy and for being prepared to give his great experience in practice in such a generous way;

His wife, Dr. Cornelia Arnoul, for the first impressions of the fascinating world of darkfield microscopy;

Dr. Klaus Karsch for being the first person to provide me with a comprehensive holistic concept which could successfully be put into practice;

Dr. Thomas Rau for many, sometimes surprising, new insights and findings;

Naturopath Willi Prigge for valuable therapy plans.

Many thanks also to Yvette Gromzig who worked with me on this book for one year, translating the German original into English. She was never satisfied before she could clearly understand what I wanted to express. Her contribution to this book has been invaluable.

And last but not least, many thanks to Monica Bryant who carried out an overall correction and checked the English terms used.

Contents

Explanation of the terms used **8**
Introduction **9**
Enderlein and his Research **12**
Summary 15
SANUM Therapy according to Enderlein in Practice **17**
Milieu Preparation **18**
Summary 18
Stimulation Therapy **19**
Stimulation Therapy Plan 22
Regulation Remedies (Fungal Isopathic Preparations) **23**
The Principles of Therapy 24
SANUVIS and CITROKEHL **26**
MUCOKEHL and NIGERSAN ATOX (EXCRETION) **26**
SANUKEHL Preparations (Haptens) **26**
Table of holistic Isopathy **28**
Supplementary Remedies 28
Application Possibilities **28**
Main Rules of SANUM Therapy according to Prof. Enderlein **30**
Summary **30**
Darkfield Microscopy and SANUM Therapy **31**
Technical requirements 31
Material needed 31
Cleaning the slides 32
Taking a blood sample 32
Results 33
Therapy Blockades **34**
Main therapy blockades in practice 34
Scars 36
The Teeth 37
Excretion **38**
Vitamin and mineral supplements **40**
Vaccinations, Drugs, Hormones **41**
SANUM Therapy, Therapeutical suggestions and cases **42**
Headaches 42
Therapy of Migraine 43
Therapy of Tinnitus 43
Cantharides plaster 44
Therapy for Influenza 45
Therapy of Chronic Sinusitis 46
Heel Autosanguis Treatment of Chronic Sinusitis 47
Nasal reflex therapy 48
Therapy of Pneumonia 53
Therapy of heart-circulatory problems 54
Therapy of Crural Ulcers 55
Therapy of recurring Urinary Tract Infection 56
Therapy of Ovarian Cysts 57
Therapy of Prostate adenoma 58
Therapy of Bechterew's disease 58
Practice case: latent Borreliosis 59
Practice case: Pancreas insufficiency 60
Intestinal *sanitation* using SANUM therapy **61**
Introduction 61

Procedure in Practice ... 62
The remedies used ... 63
The isopathic SANUM preparations for intestinal problems ... 63
Candida - a controversial topic ... 64
Nystatin - yes or no? ... 65
The diet against fungi ... 65
The plan for intestinal therapy ... 66
The plan for intestinal *sanitation* with candida fungi present ... 67
Therapy of stomach problems ... 70
Checking of the therapy results ... 70
The intestines and their psychological importance ... 70
Horvi Therapy ... 71
The unpopular subject of diet ... 71
Blood Group Diet ... 72
Water - our most important nutrient ... 72
References ... 74
Literature ... 74

Explanation of the terms used

We have our own terms in German natural health medicine and they do not always correspond to the terms used in conventional medicine. Therefore I would like to explain the terms used:

terms used in natural medicine	explanation
milieu	refers to the chemical environment within the body as the foundation for all processes of the body (thus e.g. each enzyme-process needs an exact pH.)
excretion **detoxification**	to eliminate waste products through the eliminatory pathways of the body: skin (sweat glands), kidneys, the bowels, and lungs
endobiont	primordial symbiont in the human body which Prof. Enderlein named *"endobiont"* (from the Greek "*endon*" = internal and "*bios*" = life)
endobiosis **endobiont charges**	pathogenic development of the *endobiont* causing a lot of today's illnesses
potentising	homeopathic prescription forms
initial exacerbation **healing reaction**	the disease is initially aggravated when you start therapy with natural/ homeopathic remedies. This is a desired effect.
therapy blocks or blockades	anything that hinders or prevents therapy progress
comprehensive therapy **holistic therapy**	always takes into consideration all organs of the body and in addition the personality of the patient with all their problems and possibilities
stimulation therapy	to provoke a response or reaction of the body
wheal(s), to wheal	to produce wheals by a subcutaneous injection, often used in neural therapy
neural therapy	application of specific remedies such as procaine by injection intracutaneous, subcutaneous or intra-articular to particular points. (Specific training in neural therapy is obligatory.)
intestinal *sanitation*	consists of intestinal detoxification, intestinal cleansing, balancing the intestinal flora and activating bowel movement = **establishing complete intestinal health**

Introduction

Today's medicine undoubtedly faces numerous problems. It is very successful in the areas of surgery and emergency treatment. At the same time there are obvious problems in the treatment of functional disorders and chronic diseases. Experience has shown us that the majority of patients suffer from problems in these two areas. A disadvantage of modern medicine is that it is divided into numerous specialised fields and that virtually only symptoms are treated. The whole patient with all their problems and their whole case history is unfortunately no longer taken into consideration.

In practice this means that the patient is often handed on from one specialist to the next for years or even decades. Each specialist prescribes medication without checking what medication has already been tried. The actual symptoms may disappear but they often reappear in a different form somewhere else in the body. Another specialist is then responsible for this new problem. The patient becomes increasingly dissatisfied. Eventually after years of trial and error they consult in desperation a naturopath.

If you ask the patient about previously prescribed medication the answer will often be a jumbled assortment of medication. These may work against each other; one medication neutralises the other; another increases the effect of the next; not to mention the unforeseen side effects. Nobody thinks of finding the cause of the original disease, they only treat the acute disease. On the contrary, the unfortunate patient's problems are eventually considered to be psychological.

This does not solve problems; it only helps to create new ones. Each suppression of a symptom eventually causes new symptoms. The body is trying to say that it has a problem which it cannot solve by itself. To simply suppress this symptom is wrong. This form of treatment inevitably causes acute disturbances to develop into chronic diseases. This process unwittingly starts with vaccinations; followed by countless, often unnecessary antibiotic treatments; the lax use of fever suppressants; cortisone and other strong medication; and amalgam fillings.
Medical literature offers examples of patients treated as above. Originally minimal disturbances in early childhood thus developed into more and more serious diseases in the course of their lifetime and eventually the patient ended up as a physical wreck in a wheelchair.

In this situation the SANUM therapy according to Enderlein is THE solution. Therapists who have witnessed completely different diseases, which have often troubled their patients for 10 or 20 years, being quickly and successfully treated with this therapy will agree with me. Unfortunately over the years many therapists have modified and added numerous other remedies and applications to Prof. Günther Enderlein's therapy. Thus, very little of the original, very simple practical application is left. This complicates matters for the beginner and for the therapist with little experience of this therapy.

But as is so often in life: What is good is always simple!

The aim of this book is therefore to present the SANUM therapy as a clear and simple concept easily applied in practice for all to whom the SANUM therapy is completely new or who have no deeper knowledge of this therapy. Thus, in a short time every therapist will be able to work very successfully using just a few remedies. You will soon realise that the SANUM therapy according to Enderlein is a relatively unspecific and easy to use therapy suitable for a wide variety of diseases and patients.

The SANUM therapy according to Enderlein is not just a therapy like so many others using numerous remedies and supplements such as vitamins, minerals and trace elements. Every day we are presented with new wonder cures which promise the impossible. Prof. Enderlein's philosophy was completely different. Enderlein often spoke of the so-called "whole health". And what do we do? We naturopaths, as well as conventional doctors, cheerfully treat each symptom separately. We work against all kinds of germs that we ourselves have defined as harmful and we dare to dictate how nature should behave. We know nothing or very little about our patients, their mission in life, their situation, their motivation and their real problems. Maybe the germ in question is not harmful to the patient but actually has a useful function. Who is in a position to make this decision?

According to Enderlein there is only one way to achieve full health: by creating a healthy milieu. This is done by bringing into harmony the patient's situation in life, their diet, their surroundings and their way of life. To wage a war against countless germs is wrong and can never be won. Daily experience confirms this. An example are helicobacter patients after conventional medical treatment. The supposed causative organism has disappeared but not the patient's complaints.

The aim of every therapy should be to influence the milieu so that the patient can live in harmony as far as possible with themselves and their surroundings. Then, all so-called causative organisms will disappear of their own accord. The result would be an almost perfect symbiosis with a wide range of micro-organisms without which life would not be possible. In this context the body only presents the results of countless mistakes over the years. It is only the victim. Not only the body but the whole person is ill. More correctly perhaps our era is ill.

Our diet is the most important factor for the milieu. Therefore this subject has to be discussed before beginning therapy. On the other hand changing their diet is often difficult for patients. (⇨ Diet)

The second factor, and often the most important factor, but unfortunately the most difficult in therapy is the patient's psychological state. The body often only presents symptoms when there are unresolved psychological disturbances. It would be too complicated to go into this further here. It is often fundamental and essential for the progress of the therapy to find out what the patient really wants and needs. Only this can be the aim of the therapy and not what the therapist thinks is important. Some people cannot get better because their illness is such a part of their life and they can only cope with life by being ill. It would be a great mistake to try to "heal" such a patient!

We are standing on rocky ground when we use the word "healing". I think it is a boundless presumption to call oneself a healer but unfortunately many do so every day. I believe we should modestly remain in the background. The aim of therapy should be to show the patient ways in which he can bring his whole milieu into harmony as far as possible, to improve his body's regulation ability and to activate the eliminatory pathways of the body. Thus, the organism regains its self-healing potential. The patient feels fit again, full of energy and full of life. That is all we can achieve and then only if the patient is prepared to undergo the necessary steps. It is important that the patient and their body do the work themselves. Therefore the problem should not be treated by simply prescribing medication. We should instead strive to help the organism carry out its functions by itself as nature intended.

You will really enjoy working with SANUM therapy if you observe a few basic rules. Above all you have a means of treating simply and relatively non-specifically a wide variety of diseases using very few remedies which vary very little from disease to disease. Your will be very successful, even in unexpected cases. In addition SANUM therapy is also very promising in the treatment of specific diseases. Nevertheless the milieu must always be treated first. The symptoms often already disappear during this phase.

Enderlein and his Research

Prof. Enderlein was born in 1872 in Leipzig. He studied the natural sciences, biology and zoology. At first he worked at the zoological museum in Berlin. Later he became a production manager for the SANUM company, which already existed then. At the same time he founded his own microbiological institute, where he developed unique preparations from fungi. Enderlein died in 1968 in Hamburg, 96 years old, physically weak but still with a completely clear mind.

Enderlein started his main research in 1914, the first year of World War I. He voluntarily offered the army his services as a bacteriologist, but because they could not find a doctor they engaged him as a staff-doctor. He was given a laboratory of his own and in addition he installed a private laboratory in his house in Stettin. Thus, Enderlein was given the chance and the means to carry out his research at the intensity he desired. He certainly used this opportunity, cycling every day from one laboratory to the other and he burned the midnight oil to continue his research.

Before beginning to discuss Enderlein's research at this point a short historical glance back:

About a 100 years before Enderlein a French chemist, biologist and professor of pharmacy, named *Antoine Béchamp*, had claimed:

- that all animal and plant cells contained tiny granules.
- that after the death of the host organism these did not perish.
- that from them other micro-organisms could arise.
- that these would be indestructible and eternal.
- that they would form the transition between non-living and living matter.

Béchamp called them "*microzymas*". He claimed that these microzymas could evolve into bacteria with putrefactive and fermentative properties. He deducted that diseases therefore had their origins **within the body**.

Thus, "*Pleomorphism*" was discovered and the foundation was laid from which further research could have continued, if *Louis Pasteur*, a French microbiologist had not been alive at the same time. *Pasteur* claimed:

- that all microbes, regardless of their type and species were unchangeable,
- that each type only produced one specific disease,
- that bacteria and fungi could never arise from spontaneous generation,

and above all,

- that blood and tissue are sterile in healthy conditions.

Pasteur believed that diseases had their origins in bacteria that attack the body **from the outside**. This is what conventional medicine still thinks today.

Another researcher, *Claude Bernard* (1813-1878) corrected the argument of both *Béchamp* and *Pasteur*. He said:

"No, gentlemen, the microbe is nothing, the milieu is everything."

According to a rumour, *Pasteur* said on his deathbed: "*Bernard was correct. The microbe is nothing, the milieu is everything.*"

When *Béchamp* died Enderlein was just 36 years old. He continued *Béchamp's* research and developed it further.

In 1916 Enderlein made his main discovery whilst working on typhus. He observed blood under a darkfield microscope and discovered tiny moving beings which entered into union with more highly organised bacteria. When they united they became invisible. Enderlein surmised processes whereby not higher forms as normally expected but lower forms developed. These tiny organisms which he named "*spermits*" could only be seen under a darkfield microscope but not under a light microscope. These vigorously moving *spermits* had flagella.

At the same time Enderlein had already recognised that in the blood of mammals there was always a symbiont of plant origin present. This organism occurred in different forms. Therefore, according to Enderlein, all life corresponds to a gigantic primordial symbiosis and all diseases are caused by disturbances of this primordial symbiosis.

Enderlein wrote and published over 500 scientific works, many of them on pleomorphism and symbiosis. He spent many years on specific research, examining living blood under a darkfield microscope. His main work is "*Bacteria Cyclogeny*" (Bakterien-Cyclogenie), published in 1925. Enderlein shows in this work that in the struggle for survival all species try to find a balance. Their aim is not to eliminate other species by killing or eating them but to live in harmony.

The essential works for the practitioner are the *AKMON I - III*, published from 1955 onwards. In my view, each practitioner, who is going to work with Enderlein's therapy and darkfield microscopy should read the three *AKMON* books. In the *AKMONs* you will find large parts of Enderlein's research on the primordial symbiont "*Mucor racemosus Fresen*". He called it the "*endobiont*" (from the Greek "*endon*" = internal and "*bios*" = life). In order to research this *endobiont* Enderlein continued to cultivate this fungus for decades.

<u>Summarised here important research results of Prof. Enderlein:</u>

- The cell is not the smallest living unit, the colloid is.
  Colloids are particles of a size under 0.2 µm.

- All bacteria have a nucleus or a nucleic equivalent. Enderlein called this "*mych*".

- Bacteria can multiply sexually and asexually.

  (This part of Enderlein's research was confirmed by the research of two American Nobel prize recipients 40 years later, unfortunately with no mention of Enderlein.)

- Scientific proof of the pleomorphism of microbes.
- Enderlein proved that blood is not sterile and germ-free. He claimed that there are living micro-organisms in the serum of all people and all warm-blooded animals. He called these "*endobionts*".

It is interesting that according to Enderlein's research the *endobiont* is evolving, caused by the use of artificial fertilizers; preservatives and food colourings; air pollution etc. The main reason for evolving and therefore becoming pathogenic though, is the overabundance of animal protein in our diet. According to Enderlein these causes are the main evils of mankind. In his AKMONs he compares our situation to "Pandora's box" in Greek mythology.

It is interesting that Enderlein believed, 45 years ago, that a bad diet with too much animal protein (meat, fish, eggs) and too much sugar is mainly responsible for our illnesses. Unfortunately a lot of Enderlein therapists do not like to hear this. Enderlein though, claimed this fattened the *endobiont*. He believed a lacto-vegetarian diet was optimal because milk protein can be metabolised easily without any problems. Enderlein was not only a vegetarian but also consumed mainly raw food. What would Enderlein say if he could see our diet today?

In my view, fish is preferable by far to meat or eggs. Fish are cold-blooded and therefore not *endobiont*-charged. Unlike Enderlein and many nutritionists I believe that milk and dairy products often cause many patients problems. (⇨ blood group diet)

According to Enderlein, disease always indicates a disturbance of the symbiosis. Under darkfield you can recognise this by the absence of certain growth forms of the *endobiont*, especially the absence of *diökothecits*.

<u>Enderlein claimed:</u>

"Diseases are caused by the development of the *endobiont* into higher valences (parasitic growth forms). These have their own metabolism which poisons the metabolism of the host organism."

"Cancer is a process of fermentation and putrefaction caused by a parasitic fungus and its growth forms."

In Enderlein's opinion the solution to questions on health and life processes is not to be found in medicine but only in biology:

"Medicine knows a lot about diseases but nothing about life!"

Summary

Here a summary of Prof. Enderlein's research:

- All chronic diseases are caused by one microbe. Man and all warm-blooded animals have lived in symbiosis with this microbe for millions of years. Enderlein called it the *endobiont*. We all live with it in a kind of "*primordial symbiosis*".

  In this connection it is interesting that the *primordial symbiont* is of plant origin. The *primordial symbiosis* is therefore the symbiosis of a microbe with plant origins - the *endobiont* - and the human or the animal cell. According to Enderlein the *endobiont* also forms the mitochondria and other cell organelles.

- All diseases are related to the evolution and pathogenic development of the *endobiont.*

- According to Enderlein there are two *primordial symbionts* or *endobionts*, both fungi:

  1. ***Mucor racemosus Fresen***
  2. ***Aspergillus niger van Tieghem***

- The term *cyclode* used by Enderlein (in English: cycle) covers all apathogenic and pathogenic phases of the *endobiont's* development.

  The most important phases of the *Mucor racemosus cycle* are:

  ⇨ **colloid** / **protit** (0,02 µm) or **spermit** = apathogenic
  ⇨ **chondrit** = apathogenic
  ⇨ **fibrin** = highest apathogenic stage
  ⇨ **bacteria** (*Leptotrichia buccalis*) = pathogenic
  ⇨ **fungus** (*Mucor racemosus*) = culmination = pathogenic
  ⇨ **death of the host organism ✝**
  ⇨ reversion of the endobiont to its original primitive stage

  The bacterial phase in the cycle of the *Aspergillus niger* is called *Mycobacterium tuberculosis Koch 1882.*

- The lower valences (*primitive phases*) of the *endobiont* (*protit*, *spermit*, *chondrit*, *fibrin*) are apathogenic and as symbionts are essential. They support metabolism and the body's defence system.

- The term "*cyclogeny*" means the evolution of the *endobiont* within its *Cyclode*. That means from the *protit* or *colloid* to bacteria and finally to fungi and afterwards back to *protit*.

  protit (colloid) ➔ bacteria ➔ fungi ➔ protit

- The upward development can be caused suddenly by changes in the milieu, particularly of the hydrogen potential (pH) or by medication like the widely used *Aspirin*.

- If the milieu changes favourably for the *endobiont* this microbe is able to end the symbiosis, become a parasite and so become pathogenic. The main causes for this are:
    - unhealthy diet (especially excess animal protein)
    - drugs / medication
    - environmental toxins
    - psychological reasons

  Diet is the most important reason for changes in the milieu: animal protein fattens the *endobiont*; reducing the animal protein intake is favourable for reverting the endobiont back into apathogenic primitive stages!

- If the endobiont has no possibility to evolve it is able to construct dry forms to survive. These permanent forms can tolerate a temperature of up to 310 ^{0}C (590 ^{0}F). They are responsible for all forms of sclerosis and stones in the body.

- In practice, when we talk about "*endobiosis*" according to Enderlein, we think of

  - the numerical increase and the evolution of the *endobiont* into pathogenic growth forms

  - body cells and blood affected by pathogenic growth forms of the *endobiont*.

  <u>The consequences for the organism are:</u>
  - production of too much lactic acid
  - higher blood viscosity
  - congestion and circulatory problems

  By administering low valent and apathogenic growth forms of the *endobiont* and by changing the milieu, especially the pH, it is possible to revert highly developed and pathogenic forms of the *endobiont* back into apathogenic lower staged forms as the lower valent forms fuse together with the higher forms. Thus, the symbiotic balance in the body is restored. The isopathic preparations used for this are therefore called regulators.

  This is true healing!

  It is important for our therapy to know that each growth form of the endobiont needs a particular milieu. We can influence the milieu ourselves by changing our diet or by taking suitable SANUM remedies. More will be covered in the practical part of this guide. (⇨ Milieu preparation)

- The transformation of higher valences into lower valences is accompanied by the production of toxins. This is what we call the "*healing reaction*" or the "*initial exacerbation*" of the illness. In connection with this the topic of excretion is important. If the toxins produced are not completely eliminated new *endobiont* charges will develop. (⇨ Excretion)

SANUM Therapy according to Enderlein in Practice

I have been treating patients for over 10 years using SANUM therapy. At the beginning and in the following years I attended seminars by more or less all of the most renowned Enderlein therapists in Germany. Nevertheless, after several years I still was not able to apply this therapy reasonably well or successfully. This changed after attending a seminar by the Bavarian doctor *Dr. Klaus Karsch*. For the first time I was given a comprehensive concept of Enderlein's therapy, which could be successfully put into practice. Since then, I know what to do and I have been able to work with SANUM therapy successfully. I have also been able to pass on my experiences in practice, in lectures and in seminars so that people are able to understand SANUM therapy easily.

Many therapists try to apply Enderlein's therapy or use the respective SANUM remedies in the same way as they apply other therapies. This means the patients come with a problem and they are simply given a remedy. In no way is this true Enderlein therapy. Personally I refuse to work this way. There are naturally exceptions; for example, if a patient comes with an acute problem, such as acute lumbago, this has to be dealt with first. Nevertheless, I point out to patients that this is only a short-term solution and not a real solution to their health problems at all. In this case the patients have two possibilities: either they are satisfied with the momentary success – and this is unfortunately most often the case – and they discontinue treatment, or they are prepared to continue the appropriate treatment.

SANUM therapy according to Enderlein is called *Isopathy*. For this a short explanation of the terms is necessary:

allopathy	means using foreign substances as in conventional medicine
homeopathy	means using like to treat like
isopathy	means using the same to treat the same

Isopathy means producing a symbiotic balance by reverting more highly developed pathogenic growth forms of the endobiont into apathogenic primitive forms by treating with low valent forms, so-called regulators.

SANUM therapy as a comprehensive concept consists of five steps:

1. **Preparation of the milieu**
2. **Stimulation therapy (using bacterial preparations)**
3. **Use of regulation remedies (fungal isopathic preparations)**
4. **Excretion (detoxification)**
5. **Supplementary methods or remedies**

For points 1 – 4 SANUM remedies are available. For point 5 there are certain remedies by other homeopathic and natural medicine companies which complement SANUM therapy very well, e.g. *Heel* or *Horvi*. I will return to this point later when I explain my therapy plans.

If you do not treat according to a comprehensive concept, that is, if you use SANUM remedies arbitrarily without milieu preparation, without stimulation and without checking the patient's whole situation, you will risk having to use a greater number of remedies over a longer period of time. You will cause the patient greater costs and you will rarely achieve the success that is actually possible. To spare my patient and myself these costs and the lack of success, I generally work according to a comprehensive concept. This means working with milieu preparation and stimulation therapy, apart from in the previously mentioned acute cases and even then I would subsequently recommend a comprehensive therapy.

Milieu Preparation

For me personally, the claims of *Bernard*, which Enderlein fully accepted, are fundamental to my work:

The milieu is everything, the microbe is nothing.

Therefore, it is necessary in our therapy to concentrate on the restoration of the milieu. This is often forgotten or neglected. I will try to explain in this book what in my opinion a comprehensive treatment according to Enderlein involves. You will also need to take into account a few things which at first do not seem to have anything to do with Enderlein's therapy. On the other hand, these accompanying steps can be decisive for the results and the success of the therapy.

When a new patient consults me I always start with a blood examination under a darkfield microscope to define a case history. The darkfield pictures, with extra information from the patient and an examination of their body gives me a good insight into the momentary milieu of the patient. If the milieu is not as it should be, there are suitable SANUM remedies to treat this.

The isopathic preparations for restoration of the milieu are mainly:

ALKALA N, **SANUVIS**, **CITROKEHL** and **FORMASAN**

The most important remedy in my practice is ALKALA N. I rarely begin SANUM therapy without using ALKALA N for at least two weeks. The remedies SANUVIS and CITROKEHL I only use for activation and treatment of local processes. More information on this point will follow later. FORMASAN I only use to treat specific diseases. I will also return to this point later.

Summary

- Start therapy by checking the patient's milieu by examining blood under a darkfield microscope. If necessary start therapy with a remedy which causes a light alkalisation of the patient. (SANUM pH regulating products)

- If you do not have a darkfield microscope it is advisable to always start SANUM therapy with a remedy which causes a light alkalisation of the patient. The SANUM remedy I prefer for this is **ALKALA N**. This remedy is an alkaline mixture of sodium bicarbonate, potassium bicarbonate and sodium citrate. It is excellently suited for the correction of the acid-alkaline balance in the organism. It is THE remedy for hyperacidity. By using **ALKALA N** you create a more suitable milieu for further therapy.

The patients should drink a glass of water with a level measuring spoon of **ALKALA N** daily for the 1st two weeks of therapy. They should drink 1/3 of this glass before each meal. Point out to the patient that they have to drink this glass of **ALKALA N** despite the fact that the indicator papers in the pack show a blue colour from the 2nd day onwards.

- Additional possibilities for milieu preparation using SANUM pH regulating products:

SANUVIS	(potentised L(+) lactic acid) regulates hydrogen potential (pH) and eliminates excess toxic lactic acid
CITROKEHL	(potentised citric acid) activates cell respiration (citric acid cycle) and is important for calcium metabolism
FORMASAN	(potentised formic acid) is important in uric acid, rheumatic and allergic processes

Stimulation Therapy

The second step in the course of SANUM therapy is in my view stimulation therapy. This is a fundamental part of a comprehensive therapy. Sometimes I start therapy with an intestinal *sanitation*. This entails stimulation therapy and therefore I do not need to carry out any additional stimulation therapy during further treatment. However, in the context of long-term therapy additional stimulation therapy is often necessary if no further progress is being made. It is important here, just as in any therapy, to remain flexible and to use all the possibilities which are available and not to stagnate in a rigid scheme.

Stimulation therapy causes:

- non-specific activation of the immune system
- excretion of toxins produced by bacteria as well as by the *endobiont*
- displacement of pathologic germs
- a change in and a regulation of the hydrogen potential (pH) as an ongoing milieu therapy

In my view, stimulation therapy is important to enable the body to be prepared for the subsequent therapy i.e. the actual SANUM therapy using isopathic regulation remedies. In practice we are mainly dealing with chronic diseases whereby the body often gets the problem under control without finding a true solution. A treatment of the disease in this chronic situation is impossible. This means we have to get the body out of this chronic, nominally regulated situation and to activate the disease into an almost acute state. The body will not be prepared to accept any therapy until this has been done. Therefore, with a few exceptions, stimulation therapy is always necessary in the course of SANUM therapy. Without this, most therapy efforts using SANUM therapy, particularly when treating chronic diseases, are doomed to fail.

For stimulation therapy the following SANUM bacterial preparations are available:

UTILIN, **UTILIN S**, **RECARCIN** and **LATENSIN**

<u>These isopathic bacterial preparations are:</u>

- Stimulation remedies
- Stimulation intensifying remedies
- Regulators of the acid-alkaline balance
- Mucosa remedies

At this point another principle of SANUM therapy according to Prof. Enderlein:

Work as non-specifically as possible and constantly change remedies in the course of a longer therapy.

As a rule, I always use all the remedies named above with the exception of UTILIN S but change them constantly. I do this according to the stimulation therapy plan given later. Each remedy has in addition a specific indication of its own. Besides, you can take into consideration the patient's type:

UTILIN	can be used when the type is lymphatic or rheumatic
UTILIN S	when the type is lymphatic and above all when there are diseases of the respiratory tract
RECARCIN	when there are mucosa or gland problems
LATENSIN	when the type is haematogenous and above all for all diseases of the stomach, the intestines and for tonsillitis

The stimulation remedies are called bacterial preparations, because they are produced from bacteria. All bacterial preparations are available in different potencies as ampoules, capsules, drops or suppositories. Thus, you can decide for yourself which application form best suits the disease and your patient. Sometimes it is effective to inject, sometimes it is enough to give capsules.

<u>**UTILIN**</u>	- Ampoules	4X, 6X
(*Bacillus subtilis = Hay Bacillus*)	- Capsules	4X, 6X
	- Drops	6X
	- Suppositories	6X
<u>**UTILIN S**</u>	- Ampoules	4X, 6X
(*Mycobacterium phlei*)	- Capsules	4X, 6X
	- Drops	6X
	- Suppositories	6X

RECARCIN	- Ampoules	4X, 6X
(*Bacillus firmus*)	- Capsules	4X, 6X
	- Drops	6X
	- Suppositories	6X
LATENSIN	- Ampoules	4X, 6X
(*Bacillus cereus*)	- Capsules	4X, 6X
	- Drops	6X
	- Suppositories	6X

When carrying out stimulation therapy there are specific guidelines to observe. Therefore please refer to the following plan for stimulation therapy. The aim is to cause a reaction in the patient's body. This reaction is the signal for us that the body is prepared to accept the subsequent therapy.

At this point a short explanation of the term reaction:
A reaction is any change no matter how slight in the state of health, and in the symptoms of the patient. The patient's symptoms may increase, diminish or disappear. Perhaps the patient's temperature will rise, or light symptoms of a former disease may appear, not as heavily as originally and, as a rule, easing off within a short time.

Depending on whether you are using injections or capsules you should take into consideration the following guidelines:

Always start injections with the weakest potency i.e. 6X. If the patient reacts you can start the intended therapy. The patient i.e. their body is ready. If the patient does not react, you should inject an ampoule of the potency 4X. If the patient then reacts you can start therapy.

You continue in this way. If you have not had a reaction at this point you should now change the remedy. In this case it is not necessary to begin with the potency 6X again because you have already prepared the body for the therapy with the first remedy. This means you should inject the next remedy 3 or 4 days later, and if you do not get a reaction, the third remedy 3 or 4 days after that, always using the potency 4X. And so on.

If necessary you can reduce the intervals to 2 days, or you can lengthen the intervals to a week, which is what SANUM-Kehlbeck generally suggests. I personally prefer an interval of 3-4 days.

Always take into consideration the patient's state of health, their age, and how long they have had the disease. This means that if there is a long-standing disease, or the patient is older, or in a bad state of health, you will have to treat carefully and give the patient all the time they need. If your patient is young and in a good state of health you can treat at shorter intervals.

Stimulation therapy using capsules is similar but gentler. Compared to injections capsules have less systemic effect. Therefore, it is not necessary to use the potency 6X. In this case you can always start with the concentration 4X but change the remedy frequently. Therefore you begin for instance with UTILIN 4X, then use RECARCIN 4X, and finally LATENSIN 4X. After this you begin again with UTILIN and so on. When using capsules, I generally administer them every two days.

If you are not successful in provoking a reaction according to this stimulation plan, you should look for therapy blockades (⇨ Therapy blockades). Therapy blockades are a very important topic in my practice. They are often the reason for unsuccessful therapies.

Stimulation Therapy Plan

	Injection (deep intramuscular)	**Capsules** (open & put contents under the tongue)
Start with	1 ampoule **UTILIN 6X**	1 capsule **UTILIN 4X**
if any reaction start therapy		
if no reaction, continue with 3-4 days later	1 ampoule **UTILIN 4X**	1 capsule **RECARCIN 4X**
if any reaction start therapy		
if no reaction, continue with 3-4 days later	1 ampoule **RECARCIN 4X**	1 capsule **LATENSIN 4X**
if any reaction start therapy		
if no reaction, continue with 3-4 days later	1 ampoule **LATENSIN 4X**	2 capsules **UTILIN 4X**
if any reaction start therapy		
if no reaction, continue with 3-4 days later	2 ampoules **UTILIN 4X**	2 capsules **RECARCIN 4X**
if any reaction start therapy		
if no reaction, continue with 3-4 days later	2 ampoules **RECARCIN 4X**	2 capsules **LATENSIN 4X**
if any reaction start therapy		
if no reaction, continue with 3-4 days later	2 ampoules **LATENSIN 4X**	3 capsules **UTILIN 4X**
if any reaction start therapy		
if no reaction, continue with 3-4 days later	3 ampoules **UTILIN 4X**	3 capsules **RECARCIN 4X**
if any reaction start therapy		
if no reaction, continue with 3-4 days later	3 ampoules **RECARCIN 4X**	3 capsules **LATENSIN 4X**
if any reaction start therapy		
if no reaction, continue with 3-4 days later	3 ampoules **LATENSIN 4X**	
If still no reaction, look for therapy blockades !!!		

When using ampoules always start with the potency **6X** !
When using capsules start as a rule with the potency **4X** !

Regulation Remedies (Fungal Isopathic Preparations)

Having completed the first two steps i.e. redevelopment of the milieu and stimulation therapy the actual therapy using fungal isopathic preparations or so-called regulators can now begin.

The most important fungal isopathic preparations are:

MUCOKEHL, **NIGERSAN**, **SANKOMBI**, **NOTAKEHL**, **FORTAKEHL**, **QUENTAKEHL** and **PEFRAKEHL**.

All remedies have their own specific effects which we will look at now:

1. **MUCOKEHL**

MUCOKEHL is produced from the *endobiont Mucor racemosus*. MUCOKEHL is the remedy to use in all cases involving the blood or circulatory system.

2. **NIGERSAN**

NIGERSAN is produced from the *endobiont Aspergillus niger*. NIGERSAN is the remedy to use for a tubercular constitution, for joint and bone diseases, urogenital, gland and skin problems, and for mould fungi in general.

3. **SANKOMBI**

SANKOMBI is a combination of the remedies MUCOKEHL and NIGERSAN and can be used accordingly.

4. **NOTAKEHL**

NOTAKEHL is produced from the fungus *Penicillium chrysogenum*. NOTAKEHL is the remedy to use for any kind of inflammation and for all bacterial infections. NOTAKEHL is also THE remedy for treating children.

At this point a very important comment:

Patients are often confused when they read "*Penicillium*" on the pack. They assume you are giving them antibiotics. Please point out to them that this is an ISOPATHIC remedy and not an antibiotic.

5. **FORTAKEHL**

FORTAKEHL is produced from the fungus *Penicillium roquefortii*. FORTAKEHL is the remedy to use for all stomach and intestinal problems. It is the main remedy for treating the intestinal flora.

6. **QUENTAKEHL**

QUENTAKEHL is produced from the fungus *Penicillium glabrum*. QUENTAKEHL is the remedy to use for any viral infection, and for any neuropathy, such as neuralgia or sciatica. Personally, I mainly use QUENTAKEHL for diseases where the nerves are affected.

7. **PEFRAKEHL**

PEFRAKEHL is produced from the fungus *Candida parapsilosis*. PEFRAKEHL is the remedy to use for any kind of fungal infection of the skin, intestines, or vagina.

The Principles of Therapy

If there is a superinfection, i.e. an acute infection caused by viruses, bacteria or fungi, you should treat this with the remedies available, either QUENTAKEHL, NOTAKEHL or PEFRAKEHL. This should be done first, before you use the remedies MUCOKEHL or NIGERSAN which revert the *endobiont* to an apathogenic state.

We have to deal in principle with two stages of therapy:

1. Treatment of the superinfection and
2. Reversion of the *endobiont* to an apathogenic state

Therefore MUCOKEHL and NIGERSAN can be used for two different purposes:

1. Specific use according to the disease and
2. Reversion of the *endobiont* in general

The Characteristics of MUCOKEHL

In my opinion MUCOKEHL is the most important remedy in SANUM therapy. MUCOKEHL is used in general for treating an *endobiosis* or what we call congestive diseases.

Type of patient: Patient with congestion in the whole body, generally due to eating too much animal protein, often combined with liver problems.

Typical diseases:

With MUCOKEHL you can successfully treat any disease which involves the blood and the circulation system such as: circulation disorders, hypertonia, anaemia, vein diseases, varicose veins, haemorrhoids; cardiovascular diseases e.g. thrombosis, embolism, heart attacks, TIA = transient ischaemic attacks, strokes; all wounds, haemorrhaging, crural ulcer etc.

Aim of the therapy: decongestion

The Characteristics of NIGERSAN

NIGERSAN is the second main remedy in SANUM therapy. It is used for treating a tuberculinic constitution.

Type of patient: degenerative, slim, with fine limbs, sensitive

Diseases of the tuberculinic constitution:

Lung diseases, bronchitis, asthma, arthrosis, rheumatism, Bechterew's disease, bone diseases, diseases of the lymph nodes, lupus erythematosus, diseases of the genito-urinary region and gonads, endometriosis, chronic pancreatitis, multiple sclerosis, skin problems, cysts, warts, benign and malignant tumours

Aim of the therapy: excretion

Isopathic Regulation Remedies (Fungal Preparations) - Prescription forms:

MUCOKEHL	- Ampoules	5X, 6X, 7X
(*Mucor racemosus*)	- Drops	5X
	- Tablets	5X
	- Capsules	4X
	- Suppositories	3X
	- Ointment	3X
	- Eyedrops	5X
NIGERSAN	- Ampoules	5X, 6X, 7X
(*Aspergillus niger*)	- Drops	5X
	- Tablets	5X
	- Capsules	4X
	- Suppositories	3X
SANKOMBI	- Drops	5X
(Combination of MUCOKEHL and NIGERSAN)		
NOTAKEHL	- Ampoules	5X, 6X, 7X
(*Penicillium chrysogenum*)	- Drops	5X
	- Tablets	5X
	- Capsules	4X
	- Suppositories	3X
	- Ointment	3X
FORTAKEHL	- Ampoules	5X, 6X
(*Penicillium roquefortii*)	- Drops	5X
	- Tablets	5X
	- Capsules	4X
	- Suppositories	3X
QUENTAKEHL	- Ampoules	5X, 6X
(*Penicillium glabrum*)	- Drops	5X
	- Capsules	4X
	- Suppositories	3X
PEFRAKEHL	- Ampoules	6X
(*Candida parapsilosis*)	- Drops	5X
	- Capsules	4X
	- Suppositories	3X
	- Ointment	3X
ALBICANSAN	- Ampoules	5X
(*Candida albicans*)	- Drops	5X
	- Capsules	4X
	- Suppositories	3X
	- Ointment	3X
EXMYKEHL	- Ampoules	5X
(Combination of ALBICANSAN,	- Drops	5X
PEFRAKEHL and FORTAKEHL)	- Suppositories	3X

SANUVIS and CITROKEHL

If you want a local effect of MUCOKEHL and NIGERSAN it is possible to achieve this by using additional remedies.

These remedies are:	**SANUVIS**	with	MUCOKEHL
and	**CITROKEHL**	with	NIGERSAN

SANUVIS	=	potentised L(+) lactic acid
CITROKEHL	=	potentised citric acid

Using these remedies you can influence the milieu in the area around the injection. The fungal isopathic preparation used will then have an increased efficiency in this localised area.

In addition, **SANUVIS** and **CITROKEHL** can be used in other situations either as drops or tablets.

MUCOKEHL and NIGERSAN ATOX (EXCRETION)

Sometimes when using MUCOKEHL or NIGERSAN the patient may suffer strong reactions caused by excretory products of the Endobiont. Some therapists then use MUCOKEHL or NIGERSAN ATOX (Excretion) to aid the excretory process. Both remedies are available either as ampoules or drops. The drops can be taken orally or rubbed into the flexure of the elbow.

SANUKEHL Preparations (Haptens)

Definition (*Roche Dictionary*):

"Haptens are incomplete antigens. They are responsible for the specific properties of an antigen. In contrast to a full-antigen they cannot produce an allergic reaction. Combined with a carrier-protein the hapten becomes a full-antigen."

The SANUKEHL preparations are a very effective part of SANUM therapy. The company SANUM-Kehlbeck considers them as the third "pillar" of SANUM therapy, in addition to the bacterial and fungal isopathic preparations. Before going into detail about the effects of the SANUKEHL preparations we should first look at the way antibiotics work.

According to conventional medicine antibiotics destroy existing pathogenic bacteria. Highly significant research proves that many antibiotics do not destroy bacteria but only their cell walls. Thus, so-called CWD (*cell wall deficient*) bacteria are created (review by *Lida Mattman*, former Prof. at the Wayne University, Detroit, Michigan, USA, 1993). These cannot be identified by the body's defence system and therefore are not attacked. The acute problem of a bacterial infection therefore may become a chronic problem. If an infection is treated with antibiotics often CWD-bacteria are created and these remain in the body undetected by the body's defence system.

This is where the SANUKEHL preparations (*haptens*) are effective. Haptens are able to mark CWD-bacteria of former bacterial infections and thus, these become identifiable to the body's defence system. Enderlein's therapy usually works non-specifically. However, in this situation there is a specific SANUKEHL remedy for certain specific bacteria. It is therefore necessary to know exactly which bacteria caused the original infection.

Function of the SANUKEHLs:

SANUKEHLs can

- connect with bacteria of former infections
- **mark CWD (*cell wall deficient*) bacteria**
- form antigens
- increase activity of lymphocytes
- make an immune reaction possible
- absorb toxins and antigens of germs
- prevent a strong initial exacerbation by other nosodes (reaction with antibodies of former contacts with antigens)

Use of the SANUKEHLs in practice:

- after each **use of antibiotics**
- for all **chronic diseases**
- for **therapy blockades**, e.g. caused by **cortisone** (**SANUKEHL Pseu**)
- after **Candida infections** (⇨intestinal *sanitation* / colon hydro therapy)
- for all toxicity caused by heavy metals
- for all **Neoplasm** (cancer)

If you want more information on this topic please read the comprehensive article by Dr. Peter Schneider of the company SANUM-Kehlbeck.

You often come to a point in the course of treatment where nothing seems to work. In this case it may be effective to ask the patient about former infections and to treat these using the specific SANUKEHL preparation. Thus, blockades caused by previous infections are removed. Subsequently, therapy can be successfully continued. SANUKEHL preparations are also effective when there are blockades caused by cortisone or toxic metals.

Prescription forms:
You can get the SANUKEHL preparations as ampoules or drops.

- Ampoules for subcutaneous injection, once a week, for at least 4 - 6 weeks

- Drops 10ml for oral or external application (rubbed into the skin)

Table of holistic Isopathy

Here once again a summary of the particular therapy steps and the available isopathic preparations:

Milieu-Preparation	**Stimulation Therapy** (activates leucocytes and lymphocytes)	**Isopathic Remedies** Regulation Remedies)
• **ALKALA N**	• **UTILIN**	• **MUCOKEHL**
	• **UTILIN S**	• **NIGERSAN**
• **CITROKEHL**	• **LATENSIN**	• **NOTAKEHL**
• **SANUVIS**	• **RECARCIN**	• **FORTAKEHL**
		• **QUENTAKEHL**
• **FORMASAN**	• **SANUKEHLs**	• **PEFRAKEHL**
		• **SANKOMBI**

Supplementary Remedies

- **Heel Remedies**
  - Traumeel S
  - Lymphomyosot
  - Mucosa comp.
  - Echinacea comp. S
  - Suis-Präparate
- **Horvi Remedies**
  (apply to the company Horvi for a therapy plan)
- **Vitorgan Remedies**

Application Possibilities

All isopathic fungal regulation preparations are available in many different potencies and prescription forms. Depending on the kind of application you have chosen, the remedies are available as ampoules, drops, tablets, capsules, suppositories, and sometimes also as ointments. MUCOKEHL is also available as eyedrops. SANKOMBI is only available as drops.

Depending on the disease you are treating, you can choose which form of application is most suitable. I personally believe in treating the whole person but apply the remedy as close as possible to the point where the disease is active. Thus, I generally only use MUCOKEHL injections of the concentration 5X and if possible intravenously because, as a rule, I am treating a blood disease. There are also exceptions, e.g. the treatment of a crural ulcer. In this case I inject MUCOKEHL in combination with SANUVIS locally into and around the wound.

As the stomach and the intestines are often affected by the disease too, any remedies taken orally cannot be fully absorbed and are therefore less effective. Therefore, if prescribing capsules, I do not let my patients take them orally. I ask the patient to open them and to put the contents, as in homeopathy, under their tongue or at the back of the throat. Using regulation remedies as drops I ask the patient to put a few drops on the back of their hand and then draw it into their nose. This is the fastest and the safest way for the remedy to reach the central nervous system. If the patient is suffering from genito-urinary disorders or other problems of the lower abdomen I prefer to use suppositories.

Table of application possibilities

Injections:	intramuscular, intravenous intracutaneous/intradermal (causing wheals on the skin) subcutaneous
Capsules:	orally, see below
Tablets:	orally
Drops:	- orally, see below - percutaneous i.e. rubbed into the skin - inhaled through the nose
Suppositories:	take daily using all suitable suppositories in rotation anal or vaginal

Capsules (always using all remedies in rotation):

UTILIN	**4X, 6X**	every 2 or 3 days,
UTILIN S	**4X, 6X**	on an empty stomach in the morning,
LATENSIN	**4X, 6X**	open capsule and spread contents under the tongue,
RECARCIN	**4X, 6X**	after this eat and drink nothing for 1 hour

Drops:

MUCOKEHL	**5X**	between once a day and once a week,
NIGERSAN	**5X**	on an empty stomach in the morning,
NOTAKEHL	**5X**	5 drops
PEFRAKEHL	**5X**	draw from the back of the hand into each nostril,
QUENTAKEHL	**5X**	after this eat and drink nothing for 1 hour

FORTAKEHL	**5X**	8 drops daily before breakfast put on dry bread and chew until it is liquid

Main Rules of SANUM Therapy according to Prof. Enderlein

- activate all excretion possibilities such as: intestines, breathing, skin (⇨ Excretion)
- provoke a reaction i.e. stimulation therapy using bacterial preparations according to the patient's state of health
- wait for reactions (weakened disease symptoms) ⇨ Stimulation therapy
- never interrupt a reaction with treatment (otherwise you will create new blockades)
- when you inject bacterial preparations always start with the weakest potency i.e. 6X.
- do not increase the potency or dosage unless the potency or dosage in use has no effect or has stopped being effective. Each unnecessary dose causes an increased production of toxic waste products.
- allow the body time to work especially in chronic cases
- if the symptoms start disappearing extend the therapy intervals
- repeat the therapy several times if necessary
- always vary remedies, potencies and dosages in the course of therapy
- treat children with low potencies, treat chronic diseases with high potencies
- for children from 6 months upwards use half the dosage, increase the dosage according to age, for children over 12 use the full dosage
- the older the patient and the more serious the disease
  the more carefully you have to treat them
- If you are treating a localised problem use in addition SANUVIS or CITROKEHL
- Never use MUCOKEHL or SANKOMBI on the same day as NOTAKEHL (MUCOKEHL and NOTAKEHL are antagonists, their effects will neutralise each other)

Summary

At this point, I will end my explanation of Enderlein and his therapy. Much of this information may be new to you. Those who have just heard of Enderlein for the first time, might have a problem following everything. Therefore I will not go into detail and give you further scientific terms e.g. for special growth forms of the Endobiont.
I do not intend to confuse you. I think basic knowledge is enough if you have no scientific interests in wanting to know further specific facts on this topic.

If you are further interested, I recommend the very good book *"Blood Examination in Darkfield"* by Mrs. *Dr. Maria Bleker*, a German doctor, published by Semmelweis. Besides the interesting darkfield pictures you will find a summary on Enderlein and his research. For me it is important, that *Dr. Bleker* kept as close as possible to the research of Enderlein, which unfortunately is not true of most of the publications over the last few years. For the recommended books ⇨ Literature.

I regret that many practitioners have adapted Enderlein's therapy using only some of his findings and have thus created their own form of therapy. This is not necessarily wrong in practice and may even be successful. However, in my opinion this is no longer TRUE Enderlein therapy.

Darkfield Microscopy and SANUM Therapy

According to Enderlein's therapy darkfield microscopy is important:

1. for the observation of the growth forms of the *endobiont*
2. for the observation of the state of blood cells
3. for keeping a check on the results and the success of your therapy

<u>My general opinion on the topic darkfield microscopy:</u>
I am a practicioner and it is important for me to know what clear information helps me and my patients in my daily work. I am not interested in trying to discover specific subtleties with the darkfield microscope. Therefore I always emphasise that it is not important for me to recognise the thousandth phenomenon of the erythrocytes.

With the darkfield, I try to gain information from just a tiny drop of living blood. This is not only about the whole organism but also about past diseases, acute diseases, and perhaps even about diseases which can be expected in the future. At the same time, I look for information on how to best treat the patients successfully using just a few remedies.

Technical requirements

You need a good microscope, a video camera and a good small television set. No more but also no less. There are some very expensive microscopes and also some very expensive video cameras, though I doubt whether you will achieve better results with them. There is no guarantee that you will get a better picture with a camera costing twice the amount. It is quite possible that the result is even worse. Therefore please consult an independent specialist.

I think however, that a video camera is absolutely necessary, otherwise the patients and the people accompanying them cannot see and follow what you are explaining. Of course a computer program and a monitor would be optimal. You could then store the video pictures so that you can refer to them later after having administered therapy. A further possibility is storing the pictures on video tapes, but the handling and the quality of these pictures is not satisfactory.

Material needed

You need:

- micro-slides
- cover-glasses
- immersion oil
- lancets (e.g. *Boehringer Softclix II*)

Cleaning the slides

One of the main problems in daily practice is the cleaning of the micro-slides. All available micro-slides are declared to have been thoroughly cleaned and ready for use. What this means is easy to see. The micro-slides are always dirty. In this condition they are useless for us. Possible cleaning methods involve the use of steam, washing-up liquid and alcohol. However, this does not really solve the problem.

When examined under the microscope we find that there are always contaminants, which may lead to false readings and interpretations! There is no perfect solution at the moment! We have to approach the problem and find a suitable solution.

In my opinion, the best cleaning results are achieved with hot water containing a very small amount of biological washing-up liquid. The micro-slides are then cleaned with a sponge, washed again in very hot water, and then air-dried on a rack on both sides. The micro-slides are then wiped dry using a clean non-fluffing tea towel.

Make sure that you thoroughly check every single packet of micro-slides for faults. Clean one micro-slide then by using your preferred cleaning method. A drop of spring water should then be placed on a micro-slide cleaned in this way and then be put under the microscope. You will be surprised what you see! Please be aware of the risk of interpreting results which may be caused by the micro-slide itself. I know a therapist who tried for a long time to identify darkfield phenomena as parasitic organisms, which were in fact merely pieces of fluff as a result of using cotton swabs to clean the slides.

Once the blood sample has been taken, it should immediately be placed under a cover glass to avoid unnecessary contact with air. This means that all equipment should be well prepared beforehand and be within easy reach, ready for immediate use.

The cover glasses used do not normally have to be cleaned manually, blow off any visible dust.

Taking a blood sample

Opinions also differ here. In connection with this, we should not underestimate the effect of animal protein effects. Please carry out the following experiment: make a darkfield blood test after a meal consisting only of salad and then after a meal with meat. You will clearly see the difference. Animal protein always activates the body's defence system so that general conclusions may be drawn on dietary habits. We are simply not aware of the body's reaction to meat. We just enjoy a piece of meat and take no further interest in how the body deals with it.

Animal protein always distorts the results of your blood examination!

In my opinion, blood should be taken in the morning after a light breakfast (coffee, tea, rolls, butter or margarine, and jam etc.). There should be no animal protein such as egg, cheese, sausage, or ham. In this respect butter is a fat and not a protein. Yoghurt is also allowed as it contains so little protein and this protein has been predigested by lacto bacteria.

Procedure for taking a blood sample:
With a lancet, a small prick is made on the side of the ring finger of the left hand. If your patient is left-handed, then the right hand ring finger should be used because there are fewer nerves running along the side of this finger and it is therefore less painful. Blood can also be taken from the ear lobe but then for consistency it should always be taken from the ear lobe. However, most therapists I know usually refuse to take it from the ear lobe.

I use lancets which are part of an apparatus called *Softclix* produced by the *Boehringer* company. However, I do not use the equipment itself as it does not usually work reliably, nor do I use normal lancets, as I find them too brutal. Sometimes there is too little blood, sometimes too much. The procedure using them is always uncontrolled. The procedure is very easy with the small needles that I use and I can prick the finger without trouble. There is rarely too much or too little blood.

The first drop of blood is usually wiped off as it contains cells and contaminants. The second drop of blood should go on the cover glass. No pressure should be applied to the finger to make blood appear. The patients should be told this as well, as some people start to squeeze if no blood drips out. On the other hand, the drop of blood should not be too large either, as this will distort the examination. In this case, you will have to wait a little until the bleeding eases off. (Caution: Marcumar patients !!!)

After blood has been taken a swab should be applied to the area for 1 or 2 minutes until the bleeding has stopped. No sterile swabs are required!

Results

At present I use an information sheet for the patients with pictures and explanations of the most important phenomena and a second one with several columns for the examination report. On this sheet I can register several examinations and compare the results over a longer period of time.

When a new patient consults me, I always start with a darkfield examination to define a case history. The patients appreciate this method more than building up a case history on the basis of their answers to my questions. I get the first indication by simply holding the patient's hand. Cold hands indicate poor circulation. I then ask the patient if they often have cold feet, varicose veins etc. I then explain to the patients everything I see in the darkfield and I ask them whether they suffer from the corresponding symptoms. If they cannot confirm it, then it is only a disposition. I then ask them whether there are other cases of this disease in their family (father, mother, grandparents etc.). The patients will generally confirm this. A careful and thorough examination will always enable you to find out any serious problems that the patients may have!

Darkfield microscopy is not a scientific examination method, whatever this may be. Rather it is an empirical method, meaning that the observation of a phenomenon is based on experience and not on a scientific examination.

A note should be made here concerning fungi:
You can never see fungi under darkfield! If you can see them then it is an indication of the approaching death of the patient!

Firstly, the general impression is important to me: what catches my eye. After this, I pay attention to the phenomena which are obvious. I do not search for any individual or rare phenomena which appear only occasionally. Generally speaking, I take care not to interpret something which is not completely clear. Here the greatest caution and attentiveness are necessary, e.g. because of possible contaminants on the micro-slide or the cover-glass.

In the case of doubt, I also send the patients to a doctor that I recommend for a conventional blood analysis including the hematocrit and other results.

A frequent question which arises in my seminars concerning the darkfield blood examination is: What should I do if this specific phenomenon occurs and which SANUM remedy should I use?

Answer: I never react to a phenomenon in the blood picture with one single remedy. On principle, I am not a therapist who reacts to a specific problem with one particular remedy. After having defined the patient's problems I will always first try to bring the milieu and the regulation back to normal. In our practice, the first step is frequently an intestinal *sanitation* as a primary milieu treatment. After this, that is after about three months, we look at the blood again, and on this basis we now have the possibility to work specifically on single phenomena i.e. the corresponding problems.

Therapy Blockades

Therapy blockades are disturbances of the vegetative nervous system and subsequently, disturbances in all areas regulated by this system. The effect of biological remedies and the healing process is blocked.

Main therapy blockades in practice

1. Vertebral column blockades:
   (physical blockade caused by displaced vertebra)

   Therapy: chiropractic, acupuncture and other vertebra correction methods

2. Energy blockades:
   (symptoms: cold hands, feet, belly, buttocks)

   Therapy: neural therapy, acupuncture, massage and other therapies

3. Blockades caused by conventional medicine:
   e.g. vaccinations, medication, chemotherapy, hormones etc.

   Therapy: SANUKEHLs, nosodes against the specific cause

   (A major cause is cortisone. Treat using SANUKEHL Pseu.)

4. Blockades caused by toxic metals:
   e.g. tap water, jewellery, amalgam fillings etc.

   Therapy: excretion using Spirulina algae

5. Blockades caused by underlying problems:
   e.g. scars, inflammation of tonsils, paranasal sinuses, gums etc.

   Therapy: neural therapy or other methods

6. Blockades caused by teeth:
   e.g. amalgam and other metals, even gold, in fillings,
   root-treated and other dead teeth

   Therapy:
   rectification of all dental problems (dental *sanitation*):

   - removal of amalgams
   - replacement with ceramic material. No metal, no gold, either!
   - removal of dead and root-treated teeth

Therapy blockades are an absolutely central issue and of major importance for me. Even with Enderlein's therapy, like with all other therapies, you may come to a point where nothing seems to work. You will ask yourself where you have gone wrong. You have followed my guidelines and correctly used MUCOKEHL or NIGERSAN etc. and nothing works. Then you must simply have a look for other problems which may be blocking the treatment. This often requires detective work. Finally, there may of course be psychological reasons which can block any therapy. If the patient's mind says stop or no, then nothing works! To carry on therapy in such a situation demands a high amount of skill and experience. This is really an art. You can observe this with long-term patients.

To illustrate this point, I had a young woman patient years ago. We worked intensively together for about 2 or 3 years. She came two or three times a week telling me all her problems, private as well as professional. Her condition continually fluctuated between good and bad. When one problem was solved, another one appeared. The symptoms moved from the throat to the intestines, from the intestines to the joints and eventually to the teeth. Sometimes the body leads you around for quite a while. I always like to compare this to peeling an onion. During this process, you naturally come to stages where there is no or hardly any progress.

During the patient's first consultation they should be asked to undress completely. I am sure though that most of us would not do that, nor would I. Thus, in spite of thorough questioning, we only get to know many important elements after several months, and sometimes by mere chance. Some relatively minor matter, a dead ("root-treated") tooth, chronic sinusitis or even just a scar can completely block therapy, no matter how good the therapy is. It may be a major problem to detect this, but at the same time it is also a challenge for the therapist.

In this connection, it is important whether and to what extent the patient has previously taken medicine. Thus, quite old patients who have hardly ever taken medicine in their lives, respond really fantastically. On the other hand, there are often young people who have already taken lots of medicine and are therefore difficult to treat.

A further point are blockades caused by toxic metals in teeth, in tap water, and in our food. The WHO says that 60-70% of today's illnesses are caused by toxic metals. Therefore I carry out a urine test for toxic metals with every new patient. Inorganic heavy metals are highly toxic and block physical regulation and thus biological therapies.

You will wonder now whether you really have to take all of this into account. You do not! It completely depends on the energy level of your patients. This probably is not a problem for a patient with 75% energy. The body says of course I have this and that problem but with the energy still available I can solve the problems by myself. It is quite different when the patient's energy reserve is only 10 or 20%. Then everything represents a major problem. These patients must have their teeth rectified and also have their house tested for natural radiation, electric charges, and other environmental disturbances. Even the bed must be placed in the right direction. You simply must do everything possible. The slightest disturbance is a major problem for this patient.

Often an energetic test i.e. EAV, kinesiology or using a biologic tensor (*biotensor*) also helps because we are often dealing not with material but with energy blockades.

Scars

Therapy blockades can also be caused by scars. Scars can interfere with energy flows. They send the wrong signals thus disturbing the whole system. The patients are very often aware of this, too. The scar for instance may itch when the weather changes. As is well-known, each body cell has an electrical charge. Operations disturb the electrical potential of the individual cells and the energy flow. Due to this, problems can arise in completely different body regions.

In connection with this I consider treatment by laparoscopy as particularly worrying. Formerly, a small cut was made during an appendix operation. Nowadays probes are inserted at three different places and are moved around within the whole abdomen. Many natural structures and intestinal hangings in the abdomen are thus damaged. Often, concrescence and endless pain is the consequence. I have many patients who have suffered pains in the lower abdomen ever since a laparoscopy. What is supposed to be so gentle about this method I do not know. I cannot understand why it should be necessary to penetrate the left side of the abdomen, then moving across the whole abdomen in order to carry out an appendix operation.
Sometimes I think this is just a matter of fashion. At the beginning everybody is so enthusiastic about it. A few years later we usually have to concede that it was not that ideal after all. For the sake of a smaller visible scar we run the risk of greater internal damage.

By using neural therapy and other methods, blockades caused by scars can easily be treated. For example, in neural therapy an injection is made under the upper layer of the scar and thus the electrical potential is reactivated. This procedure is repeated 2 or 3 times a week and then, if necessary, once or twice a year. In order to remove disorders caused by scars I use *procaine* 1% and *Cutis* of the Heel company. Despite claims to the contrary procaine does not cause any problems if used correctly. The documented problems with procaine in medical literature are only problems that were caused by over-dosage by dentists. To be on the safe side, a procaine reaction test should be carried out by applying a drop in the eye or by injecting a small amount subcutaneously on the forearm, or use *Lidocaine* which rarely causes problems.

Neural therapy nevertheless should not be used without having acquired the necessary knowledge in specific seminars.

The Teeth

Teeth very often present a major problem during therapy. Unfortunately, most dentists are only craftsmen and not even particularly good ones at that. Most of them have no understanding of biological therapy at all. It is a well-known fact that teeth have energetic links to all organs in the human body. They can therefore cause disturbances in these organs and block therapy.

So-called "*dead teeth*" (root-treated teeth) are in this connection a really controversial subject. The dentist speaks misleadingly about root treatment, however, after root treatment the tooth is actually dead. The root of a tooth is not treated but killed and the root channel filled with a toxic material. The consequence is always a granuloma because the body will always try to reject any dead part in the body. And this granuloma then presents a serious problem. It spreads toxins in the whole body. This has been proved by tests carried out in the USA that show a clear relation between dead teeth on certain meridians and breast cancer.

Some years ago I had an 18-year-old female patient. She suffered from constantly swollen lymph nodes and chronic sinusitis. Despite intensive treatment we did not make any real progress. By chance I saw during a consultation that one of her incisors had a narrow black edge above it. I asked her and she confirmed that she had been suffering from bacterial inflammations of this tooth for several years. In addition, the tooth was dead or, as a dentist would say, had undergone "*root treatment*".

I checked my table of tooth organ relations and found a relation between that particular tooth and the paranasal sinuses and that this tooth is considered a lymphatic regulator. Thus, the problem was clear. It was not until the dentist had solved the problem with that tooth that the other physical problems could be solved, too. Such a tooth condition can completely block any isopathic or homeopathic therapy!

I have been working as closely as possible with a dentist for several years. I test the patient's toxic metal levels and which problems are caused by this before the dentist starts treatment. Then he examines the patient and removes the parts that have to be removed, e.g. amalgam. Then he proceeds with further provisional treatment.

Then I activate the excretion of material and non-material build-ups (toxins and negative information) using nosodes, homeopathy or *Spirulina*. Finally, before the dentist completes the patient's treatment, I first test all the material used, particularly all dental glue used. In my view, only ceramic material such as porcelain should be used, therefore no gold either. There should be no metal at all in the mouth. It is not possible to use pure gold but alloys, which again can cause problems. If you need dentures later, you will then have different metals which may cause problems, too. There are always electric currents between different metals and these disturb the nervous system and the whole body. Nowadays, the technical standard of a porcelain substitute is very high with a very high durability. The best glue material from the biological point of view is dental cement.

Unfortunately, very few patients are prepared to undergo such comprehensive dental *sanitation*. Also, there is always more interest on my part to co-operate than there is on the part of the dentist.

Excretion

The body accumulates and deposits waste over the years due to bad diet, certain illnesses, metabolism problems and an insufficiency of the excretory organs. This influences the milieu, hinders regulation and is possibly toxic. In the course of a comprehensive therapy the excretory organs therefore have to be activated in order to remove this waste. There are various ways of encouraging excretion.

Listed below are my preferred methods of excretion:

Intestinal cleansing:

- **Colon hydro therapy** as a fundamental part of a comprehensive therapy
- **Enemas** (e.g. coffee enema, increases secretion of gall and pancreas)

Colon hydro therapy: In most cases I work with Colon hydro therapy (⇨ Intestinal *sanitation*) and thus achieve the best results. I use Colon hydro therapy not only for cleansing but as a basic measure in general for the redevelopment of the milieu and the regulation in the body.

Coffee enemas: For liver, gall bladder or pancreas problems coffee enemas have proved successful. Liver and gall bladder problems can be influenced positively by numerous herbal remedies. Pancreas problems such as insufficiency are quite difficult to treat, take a long time, and there are relatively few available remedies. Two of them are *Okoubaka*, a homeopathic remedy and OKOUBASAN by SANUM. Using these in combination with CITROKEHL success is possible but it is a long-term therapy. Very important is absolute alcohol abstinence. I do not use remedies to substitute the pancreas enzymes. The organ would then become even less active. Instead I try to reactivate the pancreas itself. The remedies *Okoubaka* or OKOUBASAN have been proven to activate the pancreas .

Preparation of coffee enema:

- take 3 tbs. of ground coffee
- boil up with 300ml of spring water
- boil for 5 min., let simmer for 10 mins.
- leave it for 10 mins.
- pour through a coffee filter
- make up to ¾ litre with spring water

Application:

- empty the bowels first by applying 1-2 normal water enema
- apply the coffee enema using an enema kit
- hold it for as long as possible

Fasting:

Fasting encourages a lot of healing processes and improves the quality of life in general. Fasting has a deep cleansing effect which is good for body, mind and soul. Whilst fasting the body is able to detoxify. Depending on the condition of the patient and the aim of the fasting there are several possibilities, such as fasting on herbal teas or water, fasting according to Dr. Buchinger, fasting on a higher alkaline diet or fasting on fruits. During fasting not only body waste is removed but also emotional ballast. It is therefore very important that the patient has suitable psychotherapeutic support.

Sweat bath / Salt bath:

Sweat baths are a very ancient treatment which have now become popular again in some hospitals. They cause a slight increase in body temperature and considerable excretion. Both help to activate the healing process. It is important that this is done correctly, which is only possible with help.

Prescription:

- drink 1 litre of hot lime flower tea (before, during, and after the bath)
- hot bath (as hot as possible) with 3 kg of household salt dissolved in the water
- rub with a brush (traditional Bavarian treatment!)
- lie in bed wrapped in sheets and blankets (including hands and feet)
- sweat for 2 hours (be careful with circulatory problems)

Wraps / Packs:
e.g. Potato packs (super for bronchitis!)

- cook whole potatoes in their skins and mash them
- mix with lard and wrap in a tea towel
- apply as hot as possible to the chest (be careful and test temperature with the back of the hand!)
- in addition, if needed, use a hot water bottle
- apply it for 1-2 hours to have an effect

Sitting Bath:
sitting in a bath-tub e.g. according to the following prescription

- 5 mins. in 15-25 cms. of warm water and 1 tbs. Bade-Borax
- 30 sec. cold with 2-3 crystals potassium permanganate (water should only be light pink!)

Leimbach Prescription (Heel):
The so-called Leimbach prescription using specific remedies from the Heel company is very effective for seriously ill patients, particularly for tumour patients. It works homeopathically, deep in the cellular structures, and encourages deep cellular excretion. Apply the following drops combined up to 6 times daily, over a period of 8 weeks, and then 3 times daily for a total of 3-6 months.

Prescription: Heel Galium, Psorina, Lymphomyosot, Phosphor Homaccord

Galium	remedy for detoxification, tumours, ulcers, kidney stones, and to activate non-specifically the body's defence system
Psorina	remedy for skin and mucosa problems, liver damage, and chronic illnesses
Lymphomyosot	remedy for patients with a predisposition to overactive lymphatic organs, oedema, swollen glands, fallible for infections, and chronic tonsillitis
Phophorhomaccord	remedy for infections of the respiratory tract

Cantharides plaster:

local application: tinnitus, earache, cystitis, ovarian cysts

Form of application: ⇨ Cantharides plaster

Nasal reflex therapy according to Dr. Krack:

using the available nasal reflex essential oil (re. book ⇨ Literature)

Form of application: ⇨ Nasal reflex therapy

Activation of kidney excretion:

drink a lot of special herbal teas

Other methods:

the use of cupping glasses, Baunscheidtism, the letting of blood, the use of leeches etc.

Vitamin and mineral supplements

I am not a great supporter of supplementing with vitamins and minerals just because the patient does not have the levels considered to be normal. We hardly know what the body really needs.

A remedy which I consider very important in the context of intestinal therapy is *Spirulina* as a food supplement. *Spirulina* contains about 60% vegetable protein and is therefore an exceptionally valuable supplement for our energy level. Many patients confirm again and again that they eat less and sometimes also lose weight but nevertheless have more energy with *Spirulina*. *Spirulina* combined with a further algae (*Lithothamnion calcareum*) which contains organic calcium and magnesium. I like to prescribe this when there is a lack of these minerals and for osteoporosis. However, I mainly use *Spirulina* for metal detoxification. As is well-known, algae have the ability to bind toxic metals and thus enable the body to excrete them. *Spirulina* is easily digestible. Only a few patients with extreme disturbances sometimes have problems.

If I prescribe other remedies e.g. vitamin E or selenium, then I do so only in organic form and never in a synthetic form. There are adequate test results that prove that the body cannot or can only partly assimilate inorganic and synthetic vitamins and minerals. If it cannot assimilate them, it must eliminate or deposit them. Both options present a problem. In my view these supplements can only be used if they have first passed through soil organisms and then via the roots into plant structures.

Therefore I do not appreciate either the mineral water regarded so highly only in Germany (⇨ water) nor the widely offered mineral supplements in our supermarkets.

Vaccinations, Drugs, Hormones

The first therapy blockades in our life are caused by vaccinations. Later, by conventional medicine such as cortisone or treatment using synthetic hormones in women and also by commonly used hormone plasters. In my view we handle these things far too thoughtlessly. Thus, I frequently advise women even after a combined hysterectomy and ovariectomy to switch over to plant-based remedies, such as *Remifemin* or *Klimaktoplant,* the effect of which are similar to hormone treatment. Most of them have felt better after such treatment. Apart from this, synthetic hormones present a serious environmental problem. It is well known that hormones are information carriers. They are absorbed and eliminated by the body without undergoing any change. They end up in our natural water supply and later in the food chain. It is a fact that men are becoming increasingly infertile. This is partly due to the amount of female hormones in our food.

Conventional medicine assumes that hormone substitution is always necessary when there is an insufficiency. I had a thyroidectomy nearly 20 years ago because of a lump. It is generally believed that in such a case hormone replacement is necessary for the rest of one's life. I stopped taking them after a couple of years from one day to the next because I could not understand why I should take them. A few years ago I had my thyroid gland examined by sonography. The doctor confirmed that my thyroid gland was completely normal. In an operation the thyroid gland is not completely removed because of the parathyroid glands. In time the remains of the organ can eventually regenerate to the normal size again. This was a very important experience for me. You should not always do what you are told to do without questioning it.

Many doctors frequently prescribe thyroid hormones for disturbances even if the patient has not had an operation. According to conventional medicine the patients have to take these synthetic hormones for the rest of their life. In my view this is wrong. The thyroid gland is not given the chance to regenerate itself. I think we underestimate the possibilities of our body. We should not interfere with nature too often. We interfere with the body system too light-heartedly without exactly knowing what we are doing and the body has to redress this. The hormone system in particular is a very sensitive system which is involved in all life processes. I think it is quite inadmissible to interfere with this system.

In connection with this, I would also like to mention the common use of medication for high blood pressure and for high cholesterol levels. In these cases conventional medicine works against the body which has not increased these levels without good reason. We should therefore try in such cases to search for the true causes and not just simply treat the symptoms.

SANUM Therapy: Therapeutical suggestions and cases

You will soon realise that most acute cases are quickly and easily treated using SANUM therapy. Only chronic illnesses, and older patients who do not respond to the remedies used are difficult to treat. An initial exacerbation is desired, setbacks or a standstill in the therapy are normal. Life is never straightforward but is always a process which moves up and down. If the therapy comes to a standstill, a further therapy blockade is usually the reason.

Even if a patient with multiple physical disorders who has already undergone more or less all possible treatments in the past without any success consults me, they do not present a problem. On the contrary they offer a real challenge and the possibility to prove what SANUM therapy and complementary natural treatment is able to achieve. It is also very satisfying to be able to help these people. It is easier to treat such patients rather than patients who are mainly emotionally or psychologically disturbed.

Frequently the patient comes with a particular problem. We start treatment and then after a while the patient's disorder improves. However, we are not quite content, neither the patient nor I. I then have to look for causes which are blocking the healing process. Thus, I usually start with an intestinal *sanitation.* A treatment of the paranasal sinuses follows later. In the meantime I treat with SANUKEHLs from SANUM. Subsequently I often send the patients to the dentist, if I have not already done so at the beginning. This would in my view be an ideal comprehensive treatment which can last 1 or 2 years but in the course of treatment the patient feels much better!

Each therapist treats with the tools which are at his disposal and which he masters. A colleague who uses TCM (Traditional Chinese Medicine) or classic homeopathy will try to solve the patients disorders quite differently than I would. The following therapy plans are therefore only a suggestion how to use SANUM therapy in practice successfully.

Headaches

<u>Causes for Headaches:</u>

- Genetic disposition
- Weather sensitivity
- Migraine
- Cervical spine problems
- Addictive foods (alcohol, coffee, tea, chocolate)
- Metabolic disorders
- Disorders of the endocrine system
- Intestinal problems
- Teeth problems (use of different metals, e.g. amalgam + gold!)
- Extreme temperatures
- Stress factors at work (noise, PC screen, artificial light, air-conditioning)
- Psychological problems

Headaches are normally a symptom and not an illness in itself. Therefore look for and treat underlying problems. You will find the possibilities for treating headaches under the corresponding topic.

Therapy of Migraine

Migraine therapy is a very interesting topic. A lot of people suffer from this problem. Conventional medicine often claims that nothing can be done and comforts you by saying that the disorder sometimes disappears after 60 or after the menopause for women. This of course is not very comforting for the patient if he is only 25 or 30. It is surprising how you can help these patients with neural therapy. An intestinal *sanitation* is often the best step to start therapy.

Certain patients experience an "aura". This means they feel the coming migraine attack. With these patients I arrange that they immediately come to my practice as soon as the symptoms appear. This may be on Saturday evening at 11 o'clock or even on Sunday morning at 10 o'clock. I then inject procaine subcutaneously to defined points and in addition to all pain points on the head. It is absolutely essential that you do not miss a single pain point since any single point is able to reactivate the problem completely. You therefore have to allow enough time for this treatment. As a rule, using this treatment the migraine attacks become rarer, weaker and often disappear completely after some time. You will experience that you can treat migraine very effectively in this way if no other causes in the background are responsible for the migraine, such as problems of the cervical part of the spine or menstruation problems. These would have to be treated at the same time of course.

Therapy plan: Migraine

Remedies: **UTILIN 4X**, **RECARCIN 4X**, **LATENSIN 4X**
1 capsule, twice a week, alternating the remedies

MUCOKEHL 5X + **SANUVIS**, **Traumeel S**,
procaine or **lidocaine**

additional:
- **intestinal *sanitation***
- check and treat cervical spine problems, liver and gall bladder problems and lower abdominal problems

Therapy of Tinnitus

As a rule, the therapy is successful if the noise has only just started and if you are able to influence the noise in any way. In this case you stand a good chance of being able to treat it. Any change, e.g. in pitch, the kind of noise, the volume etc. is decisive. Any change or temporary disappearance can be considered a success. If no change occurs during therapy and if the problem is long-standing it will be hard to treat it.

Remedies: **UTILIN 4X**, **RECARCIN 4X**, **LATENSIN 4X**
1 capsule twice a week, alternating the remedies

Cantharides plaster or **Cantharides ointment** behind the ear
(⇨ Cantharides plaster)

subsequently: **MUCOKEHL 5X** + **SANUVIS** + *procaine* mixed in a syringe and injected subcutaneously once a week into the mastoid points and into specific points around the ear

SANKOMBI
twice daily rubbed on the mastoid

I always use a Cantharides plaster (⇨ Cantharides plaster) for treating tinnitus according to the following plan:

On the first day you apply the plaster. On the second day remove the plaster. A blister should have formed. Draw up the contents of the blister with a syringe. Mix this with an ampoule of *Colibiogen* and inject it intramuscularly into the left or the right buttock. In addition inject an ampoule of MUCOKEHL into the mastoid. If the noise has already changed or changes the following day, you stand a good chance of success. Depending on your assessment of the situation you continue treatment.

Normally you mix one ampoule of procaine and one ampoule of MUCOKEHL together and inject it into three defined points around the ear once a week. You do this for a total of 10 weeks. During this time the noise might change, perhaps disappear and come back, or sometimes disappears completely.

If you do not want to inject, let the patient rub in some drops of SANKOMBI on the mastoid once a day.

Cantharides plaster

Cantharides are Spanish flies. They are used in an ointment and applied with a plaster. This activates excretion via the lymph system when treating tinnitus, swellings of the joints, sciatica, back problems, menstrual problems, lower abdominal problems in women etc.

Materials:	- Cantharides ointment strong - Cantharides ointment mild - wooden spatula - *Zemuko* cellulose wadding tissues 10 cm x 2 m - sterile compresses in various sizes - plaster *Leukosilk* 2.5 cm and 1.25 cm wide - zinc oxide wound powder

Prescription:	**Cantharides ointment strong**	**Cantharides ointment mild**
	Cantharidispulver 16,25	Tine cantharidis 10,0
	Ac. aceticum 1,25	Oleum arachidis 2,0
	Oleum terebint. 6,96	Adeps benzoaticum 2,0
	Cera alba 8,15	Cera flava 1,0
	Adeps benz. 9,29	Ung. molle ad 50,0

Application:	1.	according to the size of the area cut a piece of wadding tissue (maximum 5 x 5 cm)
	2.	spread the *Cantharides ointment "strong"* approx. 1 mm thick on the tissue and on top of that a thin layer of the *Cantharides ointment "mild".*
	3.	apply it to the desired area, attach it well with an adhesive plaster and cover it with more wadding tissue.
	4.	remove the plaster after 24 hrs., draw the liquid from the blister formed with a needle and syringe, mix this with 1 ampoule of *Colibiogen* or *Lymphomyosot* and inject intramuscularly.
	5.	remove the blister and the affected skin as far as possible, apply a sterile compress and wadding tissue.
		Change as frequently as needed.

Therapy for Influenza

1st day: 1 amp. **NOTAKEHL 5X** + 1 amp. **Heel Engystol N**

2nd day: 1 amp. **NOTAKEHL 5X** + 1 amp. **Heel Traumeel S**

3rd day: break

4th day: 1 amp. **MUCOKEHL 5X** + 1 amp. **Heel Engystol N**

5th day: break

6th day: 1 amp. **MUCOKEHL 5X** + 1 amp. **Heel Traumeel S**

all remedies mixed in a syringe and injected intravenously

after this: continue treatment in the same or in an adapted form every 3 to 4 days

complementary remedies: **Heel Echinacea comp.**, **Mucosa comp.**, **Lymphomyosot**, **Coenzyme**

When treating children you can use the same remedies as drops or tablets!
(1 x 8 drops or 1 - 2 tablets daily)

Therapy of Chronic Sinusitis

I consider this subject to be very important. I estimate that two-thirds of the population suffer from chronic sinusitis, in most cases as a result of numerous incompletely healed sinusitis infections or because of sinusitis that has been treated with antibiotics for years or decades. Many patients have become so accustomed to their problem, that they accept it as normal and do not even mention it of their own accord during their first consultation. The body has adjusted to this chronic problem but has not resolved it. When questioning the patients for their case history I never forget to ask whether they suffer from sinus problems.

Each minor cold can lead to chronic sinusitis caused by a superinfection. Using the wrong remedies, especially antibiotics, increases this risk. Each chronic process in the body occupies the body's defence system and therefore represents a therapy blockade. Since chronic sinusitis occupies the body's defence system permanently the latter is no longer fully available for other needs. Particularly older patients often have other chronic illnesses in addition to sinusitis and the regulation ability of their body is handicapped greatly by these multiple disorders. Often the body then rarely allows any therapy efforts. We may therefore have to deal with serious therapy blockades.

Therapy plan: Chronic Sinusitis

Remedies:

Utilin 4X, **Recarcin 4X**, **Latensin 4X**
1 capsule twice a week, alternating the remedies

Nigersan 5X, **Sankombi**, **Notakehl 5X**
5 drops drawn into each nostril, alternating the remedies daily

optional:

twice a week according to the plan:

Autoblood injections with Heel remedies:
Traumeel S, **Mucosa comp.**, **Lymphomyosot**, **Sinusitis Nosode**
twice a week (⇨ Autosanguis Heel) or

Autoblood with **Colibiogen** injections or **Colibiogen** drops

additional:

Nasal reflex therapy according to Dr. Krack
Once or twice a week (⇨ Nasal reflex therapy)

Urine therapy with cotton buds daily if necessary
(⇨ Nasal reflex therapy)

Intestinal *sanitation* according to the plan
(Paranasal sinuses and teeth are a favoured location for toxins that the intestines cannot deal with!)

optional acc. to Dr. Rau: Patients lay on their back, with the head lower than the body

1 amp. **NOTAKEHL 5X** + **Heel Traumeel S** + **Heel Mucosa comp.**
fill up with sodium chloride to 10ml

5ml with a syringe without a needle or a pipette into each nostril, i.e. to each blocked passage

after 5 -10 mins.:
1 amp. **SANKOMBI** + **FORMASAN** + **Heel Coenzyme comp.**
in the same way

Heel Autosanguis Treatment of Chronic Sinusitis

I favour the *Heel Autosanguis* treatment if the patient is suffering from chronic sinusitis. This is an autoblood therapy with homeopathic remedies from the *Heel* company according to *Dr. Reckeweg*, twice a week, for 10 weeks.

The treatment is as follows:

First step:
Draw up an ampoule *Traumeel S*. Insert the needle into the vein of the arm. Then you draw about up 0.5 - 1ml of blood from the vein and subsequently inject both together into the vein leaving about 0.1ml in the ampoule.

Second step:
Draw up 1 ampoule *Heel Mucosa comp.* with the same syringe, then 1ml of air and shake all of this together ten times. After having removed the air the mixed substances are injected intramuscularly into the right buttock leaving again 0.1ml in the syringe.

Third step:
Draw up the remaining two *Heel* ampoules *Sinusitis Nosode* and *Lymphomyosot*, proceed as in step 2 and inject this into the left buttock.

Thus, with this treatment we achieve a stimulation of the body in three different places.

Therapy plan Heel Autosanguis

1.	Draw up an ampoule **Heel Traumeel S**. Insert the needle into the vein of the arm. Then you draw about 0.5 - 1ml of blood from the vein and subsequently inject both together into the vein, leaving about 0.1ml in the ampoule.

2.	Draw up 1 amp. **Heel Mucosa comp.** with the same syringe, then 1ml of air and shake all this together ten times. After having removed the air the combined remedies are injected intramuscular into the right buttock, leaving again about 0.1ml in the syringe.

3.	Draw up the remaining two Heel ampoules **Sinusitis Nosode** and **Lymphomyosot**, proceed as in step 2 and inject this into the left buttock.

in addition: **Heel Euphorbium comp. S** nose drop spray

In addition to this medical therapy I treat with the Nasal reflex therapy according to *Dr. Krack* (⇨ Nasal reflex therapy). I strongly recommend this treatment. If the problem has not been solved by the treatment so far, there are further possibilities such as the therapy according to *Dr. Rau*. Your aim should always be to stimulate the body by changing methods again and again to prompt the body to work on the existing chronic problem. You should consequently continue treatment until the existing problem is solved completely.

Nasal reflex therapy

Nasal reflex therapy according to Dr. Niels Krack can be used to treat many physical problems by stimulating the reflex zones in the nose. If you want to find out more about all the possibilities of this therapy please read the book by Dr. Krack (⇨ Literature). I will concentrate here on the treatment of sinusitis using Nasal reflex therapy because we have successfully used this therapy to treat this problem for many years now. Before you start the treatment of sinusitis it is advisable to read the book. The book offers extensive information on all the therapeutic possibilities but also offers an insight to an era in medicine which has fortunately passed. Several formulations are amusing, others rather frightening, such as: "The sick person sits on a chair, calm and composed and completely at the doctor's mercy. The necessary orders are given." Or in another part: "Whilst breaking the resistance of the sick person in this way....."

Unfortunately horror stories are still being spread about this useful treatment, which if applied correctly does not cause any problems. As in most cases, these are unfounded rumours. They are often the result of unqualified information by therapists who have never used this beneficial therapy. (This is also true for colon hydro therapy.) Any therapy is dangerous when used incorrectly. Therefore you should use Nasal reflex therapy carefully. I have never experienced any problems and have been using Nasal reflex therapy for more than 10 years now.

Using Nasal reflex therapy you can successfully treat chronic sinusitis. The treatment and the special combination of essential oils helps to loosen any existing incrustation. The mucosa in the nose and the openings of the paranasal sinuses are opened up again. Often patients experience instant relief after the first treatment. I do not know any other therapy method which is able to achieve this result. In addition you can prevent new infections.

Very important for therapy is the connection between the intestines, paranasal sinuses and teeth. Thus, you often find chronic sinusitis if you have a patient with intestinal disorders. In this case you cannot treat the intestinal problems successfully until you have solved the sinusitis problem.

When carrying out Nasal reflex therapy it is absolutely important that you radiate calmness and confidence. A lot of patients suffering from chronic paranasal problems are so sensitive around their nose that they are not prepared to let you do anything in this area. Therefore do not wave the metal rod around in front of the patient's eyes. This might frighten the patient. Calmly and clearly explain the treatment to the patient. Thus, before starting treatment I show the patient a little sketch of the inside of the nose and I explain what I intend to do.

At the same time I try to make them feel relaxed by pointing out that

- I will carry out the treatment very carefully and not use any force.
- I will immediately be aware if it is painful and react accordingly.
- I will immediately be aware when they have to sneeze and that I will draw the rod out of the nose in time.

Especially the last point is important for most patients. You should therefore not omit to mention it.

As a rule I treat patients twice a week for a few weeks. I do not think it is necessary or beneficial to treat more frequently because this would overstimulate the nasal mucosa. When treating long-standing chronic sinusitis I subsequently prescribe nasal reflex oil so that the patients can carry out the treatment themselves at home twice a week. The patients can use normal cotton buds. In rare cases, when the nose of the patient is very small and narrow I give them a metal rod, explaining carefully how to use it. The whole treatment should be continued until the problem is completely solved, i.e. when the paranasal situation is completely free of symptoms.

An interesting complementary treatment to Nasal reflex therapy using essential Nasal reflex oil is Nasal reflex therapy using the patient's own urine, providing that the patient does not suffer from a urinary tract infection. It would logically not be wise to spread the bacteria from the urinary tract to the nose. For urine treatment, you use the first urine of the day, which contains the most important substances. Urine therapy is in principle stimulation therapy. It is therefore suitable for influencing chronic problems positively. I ask the patients to treat themselves twice a week with oil and on the remaining days with urine until the problem has disappeared completely.

It is important to tell the patients that they should use Nasal reflex therapy in the future after every minor cold as soon as the swelling of the mucosa has receded and that they should continue treatment until the nose is completely free of symptoms. Using this treatment it is possible to successfully prevent an infection of the paranasal sinuses.

<u>Practice:</u> Nasal reflex therapy of Chronic Sinusitis

<u>Material:</u>

- metal swab rod - Art. Nr. 36052
  (Methatec GmbH, Postfach 9027, D-89087 Neu-Ulm,
  Tel. 0800-3833830, Fax 0800-3833831)
- cotton wool (acc. to Dr. Bruns)
- nasal reflex oil mite (Wecoton)
- vaseline
- paper handkerchiefs

<u>1st step:</u>

1. A little bit of cotton wool should be carefully pulled apart to make a fine cotton pad. (size: approx. 3 x 1,5cm) This pad should be wound on the metal rod firmly by strong pressure between the thumb and forefinger of your left hand and by turning the metal rod with your right hand. The tissue should be approx. 0,5cm longer at the top than the rod to protect the mucosa in the nose.

   <u>Please note:</u>
   This swab produced on the metal rod should be firmly attached to the rod. There should be no danger of it coming loose and falling off! If the swab nevertheless does come apart in the nose it has to be removed at once using a nasal speculum. Otherwise there is a risk of it being aspirated into the lungs!!!

2. The swab should then be moistened with a few drops of *Nasal reflex oil*. You can also dip the swab into the bottle with the oil. In this case it is necessary to use a separate bottle for each patient.

<u>Therapy:</u>

1. The patient sits on a normal chair.

2. You stand behind the chair, give the patient a paper handkerchief and take the patient's right hand with your left hand. Then the patient lays his head on your left arm and on your chest. He should feel safe and confident in this position. On the other hand you will immediately sense any tension that the patient may feel and can then react accordingly.

   This moment is decisive for further treatment: the patient senses at once if you are tense. In this case he will react with tension too, perhaps even with fear! On the other hand the patient is understandably tense but this tension will dissolve if you radiate calmness and confidence.

3. Quietly ask the patient to breathe through his mouth.

4. Ask the patient on which side of his nose he has more problems. Then always begin by treating the better side.

5. Hold the prepared metal rod lightly and loosely between the thumb and forefinger. This gives you the best feeling. (Do not hold the rod in a cramped manner! The patient would feel this at once and would then not be prepared to continue treatment.)

6. Now introduce the rod, moistened with oil, into the middle passage of the nose (position 1). If the patient holds his head upright the direction is normally horizontal. Carefully twist the rod to and fro whenever you feel any resistance. You will realise immediately when the passage ends and you have reached the free area in the throat. After this you draw the rod back slowly always twisting it slightly.

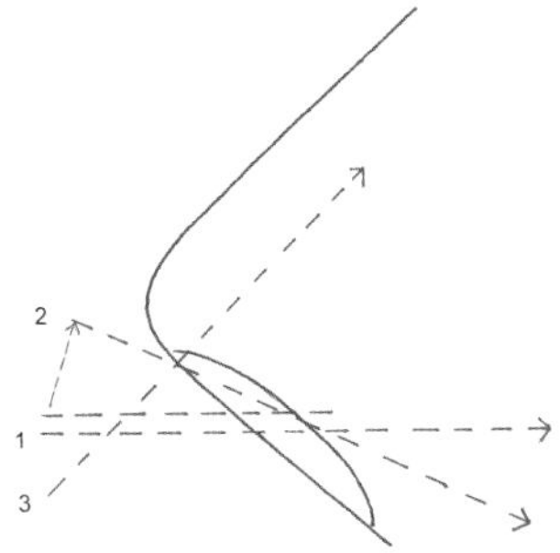

Diagram to show the three positions used for Nasal reflex therapy

At all narrow points you carry out a gentle massage by twisting the rod. After this you allow the patient a moment to relax. Then you treat the lower nasal passage (position 2) in the same way. This passage is most important because it has numerous reflex zones related to the lower abdomen, stomach, intestines, liver, pancreas, head, eyes, ears and respiratory organs. Any disturbances in these organs can therefore be treated by stimulation of the nasal reflex zones. Therefore take the time you need for the treatment of the lower nasal passage. You will find the direction for the rod if you introduce it into the nose slightly, then lift it a bit at the end and push it slowly and carefully in the new direction into the nose. This passage also ends in the free area in the throat.

Finally you introduce the rod into the upper nasal passage (position 3). At the end you will feel an obvious resistance. The direction is parallel to the bridge of the nose. The patient often reacts to the introduction into this last passage with a strong tickling and sneezing sensation. It is important that if the patient needs to sneeze you are ready to withdraw the rod quickly.

7. Sneezing now or later is therapeutically desired. It releases blockades in the body and emotional blockades too. In many cases sneezing is a very important experience for the patient.

8. After having completed the previous steps you prepare the rod with a new swab and then treat the other side of the nose in the same way.

9. When you have finished therapy prepare the rod with a new swab and vaseline and with this treat all 6 nasal passages for a short time. This will calm down the mucosa and the patient usually finds this soothing.

additional: **Nasal reflex ointment**
(vaseline mixed with a few drops nasal reflex oil) so that the patient can carry out treatment by themselves using normal cotton buds.

Luffa nosespray DHU
This spray is very soothing after Nasal reflex therapy and if necessary in the intervals between treatment.

Practice case: Chronic Sinusitis

Patient, male, 47, chronic insomnia for 10-15 years; pressure in head; chronic sinusitis, feeling that something is running down the back of the throat, followed by flatulence; stool irregularity and alternately diarrhoea and constipation

Darkfield: Intestinal rolls ("money rolls"), high activity of symprotits, numerous small laden, granulocytes

Therapy: One session of **Nasal reflex therapy** according to Dr. Krack:
patient had to sneeze vigorously and repeatedly for the 1st time in years and immediately felt a great improvement.

Prescription: **UTILIN 4X**, **RECARCIN 4X**, **LATENSIN 4X**
1 capsule twice a week, alternating the remedies

Intestinal *sanitation* according to the plan:
8 x Colon hydro therapy, **SANUM** remedies, **Mutaflor**

Change the diet according to the blood group:
(type 0 = no dairy products!)

Nasal reflex therapy with Nasal reflex essential oil "mite" (once a week) and the patient's **own urine** applied with cotton buds (daily)
(⇨ Nasal reflex therapy)

The patient felt much better, slept better, but still occasionally suffered from secretions running down the back of the throat followed by flatulence.

Therapy: **Heel Autosanguis** (10 x) with **Traumeel S** (intravenous), **Mucosa comp.**, **Lymphomyosot**, **Sinusitis Nosode** (intramuscular)(⇨ Autosanguis Heel)

Further improvement but still some remaining symptoms. A further anamnesis brought to light previous problems: middle ear infection, tonsillitis

Therapy: Injection intramuscular: **SANUKEHL Strep** (1 x)
according to a laboratory test of a swab taken from the patient's mucosa of the throat

according to **Dr. Rau:**
Patients lay on their back, the head lower than the body

1 amp. **NOTAKEHL 5X** + **Traumeel S** + **Mucosa comp.**
fill up with sodium chloride to 10ml

5ml with a syringe without a needle or with a pipette into each nostril, i.e. to each blocked passage in the nose

after 5 -10 mins. in the same form:
SANKOMBI + **FORMASAN** + **Heel Coenzyme comp.**

The patient experienced great improvement but was still not completely satisfied. I then proposed a rectification of dental problems. (removal of amalgam fillings!)

Unfortunately the patient did not return after this recommendation.

Therapy of Pneumonia

Here is the plan for treatment. Please, believe me: this is very effective; there is no need for antibiotics! Unlike with antibiotics you actually achieve a true cure. The bacteria do not go underground where they continue to do mischief as cell wall deficient (CWD) bacteria and by so doing cause chronic problems. Of course the patients would prefer an injection that makes the problem disappear instantaneously. Unfortunately, or perhaps fortunately, it is not possible to rectify years or decades of incorrect treatment with just an injection. Therefore you must make the following advice clear to the patient: either we will do it properly once and for all or the problem will remain throughout their lifetime and even become worse.

If you treat your patients using SANUM therapy and manage to avoid any use of antibiotics, you can stabilise their overall condition within 2 or 3 years. Patients with a weak immune defence, who previously had flu or bronchitis five times a year sometimes never have another serious infection. Numerous patients whom I have treated for a variety of infections over the years have never needed antibiotics again. Many people today react allergically to antibiotics. One common side-effect is diarrhoea, which can fast become a serious problem especially for older patients with a cardiac insufficiency.

The remedy NOTAKEHL in the following plan works against the actual pathogenic germs, that is, the superinfection. MUCOKEHL treats the *endobiont*, the *Mucor racemosus*, which is always active in the background. The real aim of each therapy is to return the *endobiosis* to the original apathogenic state. Therefore we have to use both remedies ONE AFTER THE OTHER.

Please remember: do not use MUCOKEHL and NOTAKEHL on the same day as they neutralise each other.

Therapy plan: **Pneumonia**

Remedies			Complementary Remedies / Methods
1st day:	**NOTAKEHL 5X** **Engystol N** **Pulmo suis injeel**	mixed injection 1 amp. of each intravenous	**Heel mixed injection:** **Echinacea comp.** **Mucosa comp.** **Lymphomyosot** **Coenzyme comp.**
and	**NOTAKEHL 5X** **Traumeel S** **Pulmo suis injeel**	mixed injection 1 amp. of each to produce sub-costal wheals	**Neural therapy:** **procaine** or **lidocaine** Subcostal to produce wheals paravertebral **Baunscheidtism**
2nd day:	continue with the same injections		
3rd day:	break		
4th day:	**MUCOKEHL 5X** **Engystol N**	mixed injection 1 amp. of each intravenous	
5th day:	break		
6th day:	**MUCOKEHL 5X** **Traumeel S**	mixed injection 1 amp. of each intravenous	
9th day:	**MUCOKEHL 5X** **Engystol N**	mixed injection 1 amp. of each intravenous	
If necessary continue or repeat therapy in the same or in an adapted form.			

Therapy of heart-circulatory problems

Remedies: mixed injection of **MUCOKEHL 5X** and **NIGERSAN 5X** intravenous once a week for 10 weeks

sometimes combined with **Crataegus Cor Wala** or **Cralonin Heel**

Wala and **Heel** remedies are suitable for complementing SANUM therapy

Therapy of Crural Ulcers

If you have a patient with a small open sore on the lower leg, e.g. after an injury from a blackberry bush, which does not want to heal you will solve this quite simply with 4 or 5 MUCOKEHL injections. You inject around the wound and also into it directly. In addition, you prescribe MUCOKEHL ointment.

Often you will have patients who have had the problem for years and nobody has been able to help them. The problem is also that conventional medicine generally tries to close the hole. Of course that is a solution but not a cure. It is wrong to simply try to close the wound. It must be healed from the inside!

Patients at an advanced stage, I first send to a vascular specialist to have their blood circulation situation clarified. You can rarely treat serious arterial circulatory disorders with natural health remedies. In this case an operation is often unavoidable.

My experience has proved that you will have great difficulties with patients suffering from obesity, diabetes or other metabolic disorders if you are unable to successfully influence the complete situation positively.

For example, I had a female patient at an advanced stage of a crural ulcer. Her fasting blood sugars were permanently at 120-140. Her doctor did not think this needed treatment. That might be true in general but not in this particular case with these symptoms. I therefore arranged for her increased blood sugar level to be treated. We would not have had any success in our treatment of the crural ulcer if this metabolic disorder had not been corrected.

<u>Therapy plan:</u> **Crural Ulcer**

Remedies	Complementary Remedies / Methods
<u>1st therapy using injections:</u> **MUCOKEHL 5X** and **SANUVIS** + **procaine 1%** 1 ampoule once a week for 10 weeks by intracutaneous injection around the affected area, if possible into the open area too! <u>optional between the above injections:</u> **NOTAKEHL 5X** + **procaine 1%** **PEFRAKEHL 5X** + **procaine 1%** **QUENTAKEHL 5X** + **procaine 1%** **MUCOKEHL 3X** ointment	**Test blood sugar!** **MUCOKEHL 3X** ointment **NOTAKEHL 3X** ointment alternating remedies daily **Bach Rescue** ointment **Traumeel S** ointment **Tea tree hydrolate** apply to affected area **Honey** (fluid quality!) apply to affected area **Curd wraps**

Remedies	Complementary Remedies / Methods
<u>2nd therapy without injections:</u>	<u>Complementary steps:</u>
MUCOKEHL 5X drops **NOTAKEHL 5X** drops **PEFRAKEHL 5X** drops	**change diet** (higher alkaline diet, reduce animal protein)
daily around the affected area	**reduce weight**
SANKOMBI draw 5 drops daily from the back of your hand into each nostril	**Intestinal *sanitation*** ***Sanitation* of the teeth**
MUCOKEHL 3X ointment	**Excretion of toxic metals**

Therapy of recurring Urinary Tract Infection

Listed are various options for the treatment of the above which can be used singly or in rotation according to the illness you are treating and depending on how long the illness has existed:

<u>1st Therapy:</u>	1st day eat dry bread only. Drink nothing! From the 2nd day onwards drink a lot!	
	UTILIN 4X, **RECARCIN 4X**, **LATENSIN 4X**	1 capsule twice a week alternating
	NOTAKEHL 3X, **EXMYKEHL 3X**	1 suppository daily alternating applied anal or vaginal
<u>2nd Therapy:</u>	**Waag Bomb** (according to Dr. Waag)	twice a week for 3 weeks
	NOTAKEHL 5X, **PEFRAKEHL 5X**, **SANUVIS**	1 ampoule of each mixed in a syringe and injected intra-muscularly into the left buttock
	FORMASAN	1 ampoule intramuscularly into the right buttock
<u>3rd Therapy:</u>	**Neural therapy**	1 finger above symphysis prod-uce a wheal with **procaine 1%**
	NOTAKEHL 5X, **Traumeel S**, **Echinacea comp. Heel**	then inject 1 ampoule of each remedy mixed in a syringe with a dental needle into the bladder

additional: **UTILIN 4X**, **PEFRAKEHL 5X**, **NIGERSAN 5X** — or other SANUM remedies according to a test*

additional: **Canephron** coated tablets — 3 x 2 daily

vaginal rinse — with Tea tree lotion (diluted!)

Intestinal *sanitation*!!!

(before the discovery of antibiotics it was well known that bladder infections are mainly caused by coli bacteria.)

* There are several test procedures. In my practice I test the suitable remedies in specific situations using a biotensor.

When treating an acute infection with severe pains inject daily on the first 3 days into the bladder, sometimes only every second day if the patient is very sensitive. According to my experience the pains lessen notably after the 1st injection! Then inject intramuscular twice a week for 4 - 6 weeks extending the intervals to once a week for another 4 - 6 weeks. If necessary continue therapy.

In my experience the illness recurs at ever greater intervals and the symptoms weaken. Treat until the problem is finally solved!

Injections into the bladder do not cause any problems when carried out correctly according to the rules of neural therapy. Please note that strong emotional reactions are possible. For example, I had a young female patient. She was greatly disturbed after the injection. I asked her if she suffered from pains, but she said no. She was not prepared or able to speak about the problem. I was glad that her friend had accompanied her. It could have become a difficult situation for me. Please make sure there is an assistant present when you administer an injection into the bladder!

Therapy of Ovarian Cysts

Remedies: **UTILIN 4X**, **RECARCIN 4X**, **LATENSIN 4X**
1 capsule twice a week alternating the remedies

NIGERSAN 3X, **MUCOKEHL 3X**, **NOTAKEHL 3X**, **EXMYKEHL 3X**
1 suppository daily alternating the remedies

optional:
- **Cantharides plaster** on the symphysis (⇨ Cantharides plaster)
- **Neural therapy**
- **Horvi therapy** (please request a therapy plan before treatment!)

after this: continue or repeat treatment in the same or an adapted form

Therapy of Prostate adenoma

Remedies: **UTILIN 4X, RECARCIN 4X, LATENSIN 4X**
1 capsule twice a week alternating the remedies

NIGERSAN 3X, MUCOKEHL 3X, NOTAKEHL 3X, EXMYKEHL 3X
1 suppository daily alternating the remedies

optional:
- **Cantharides plaster** on the symphysis (⇨ Cantharides plaster)
- **Neural therapy**
- **Horvi therapy** (please request a therapy plan before treatment!)

after this: continue or repeat treatment in the same or an adapted form

Therapy of Bechterew's disease

SANUM therapy according to Prof. Enderlein when treating Bechterew's disease is often very successful. Important is a consequent long-term use of numerous remedies often applied by neural therapy methods. It is normally not possible to cure the illness with this therapy, but depending on the stage of the disease you can at least relieve the pain, maintain as much mobility as possible and stabilise the disease so that no further exacerbation is to be expected.

Practice case: Bechterew's disease

Patient, male (33), Bechterew's disease, in severe pain, and stiffening of the lower spine. The therapy according to the following plan was successful in reducing his pain greatly and preventing further progress of the illness. The patient could ride his horse again and go skiing, which was a major improvement to the quality of his life.

Therapy plan: Bechterew's disease

Therapy 1: **MUCOKEHL 5X, QUENTAKEHL 5X, SANUVIS**

1 ampoule of each in a combined injection with 5ml procaine 1% producing paravertebral wheals to vertebra C1 - L5

alternating weekly with a combined injection of 1 ampoule of each of the following remedies and 5ml procaine 1%

NIGERSAN 5X, NOTAKEHL 5X, CITROKEHL

Therapy 2: according to Dr. Wolfgang Köstler (⇨ SANUM-Post No. 4) for 6 weeks

LATENSIN 4X 4 - 5 ampoules

These are drawn up and injected intramuscularly in one treatment

Please note: it is painful and strong reactions are to be expected!

I therefore only administer this injection following long-term treatment with SANUM remedies.

To keep up a stimulation it is advisable to alternate between therapy 1 and 2 if you carry out a long-term therapy.

additional:	**Coenzyme comp.** Heel	1 ampoule once a week intramuscular
	Phlogenzym Mucos	3 tablets twice daily
optional:	**Use of cupping glasses**	
	Baunscheidtism	
	Intestinal *sanitation*!!!	
after this:	continue or repeat in the same or in an adapted form	

Practice case: latent Borreliosis

Patient, female, 18, chronic tendovaginitis in both lower arms after a tick bite 5 years previously, headaches, chronic tiredness, rheumatoid factors, intestinal problems, paranasal problems, previously recurring tonsillitis. Severe pain did not enable the patient to do schoolwork or play the piano. Conventional treatment had had no success.

Darkfield: Intestinal rolls ("money rolls"), "lemons" = liver problems, "fried eggs" = less energy, filits, rheumatic disposition, numerous small laden granulocytes

Therapy: **Intestinal *sanitation*** according to the plan:
8 x Colon hydro therapy, **SANUM** remedies, **Mutaflor**

Change diet according to the blood group: type 0 = no dairy products!

Nasal reflex therapy with Nasal reflex essential oil "mite"
(once a week) + her own urine applied with cotton buds (daily)
(⇨ Nasal reflex therapy)

Injection once a week intramuscular:
Staufen Borreliose potentising sequence (NL-Holomed)

Injection intramuscular (1 x): **SANUKEHL Brucel**
(⇨ SANUM-Post No. 43)

The patient was a completely different person, enthusiastic, hardly any symptoms, and could write and play the piano again! Treatment was continued. Don't stop treatment too soon!!!

Practice case: Pancreas insufficiency

Patient, female, 54

Remedies:	**UTILIN 4X, RECARCIN 4X, LATENSIN 4X** 1 capsule twice a week alternating remedies for 6 - 8 weeks
	OKOUBASAN 3 times daily 1-2 tablets
	CITROKEHL 3 times daily 1-2 tablets
additional:	**Colon hydro therapy**

Laboratory	Elastase-1	01.12.1999	164 µg / g stool
Test:		05.02.2001	240 µg / g stool

normal levels:	normal	> 200 µg / g stool
	light / medium insufficiency:	100 - 200 µg / g stool
	severe insufficiency:	< 100 µg / g stool

Another patient's test results developed as following:

Elastase-1	01.08.2000	50 µg / g stool
	15.01.2001	78 µg / g stool

If you have reason to believe there is a pancreas insufficiency you can get a good insight into the pancreas function by testing the enzyme Elastase-1 in a stool examination.

Intestinal *sanitation* using SANUM therapy

Intestinal *sanitation* is a comprehensive treatment of the intestines. The aim is to heal all functional intestinal disorders, to restore the intestinal mucosa and to reinstate a natural and healthy intestinal flora.

Introduction

On this subject and the relevant therapies there are many different and often contradictory opinions. Even many Enderleinian therapists underestimate the importance of intestinal therapy. Only after treating numerous patients over a long period of time can we realise how important a role the intestines play in our life. For me the intestines are of major importance. And I do not stand alone in believing this, either. The Russian Nobel prize winner *Metschnikoff* claimed: "*Death is sitting in the intestines!*" Many older patients confirm again and again that their mother had always paid attention to a regular bowel function. This knowledge is all but lost today.

It is indisputable that the intestines as a whole represent a major organ system in the body. The decision concerning which substances are absorbed and which substances are excreted is made in the intestines. The intestines are basically responsible with the help of intestinal bacteria for the regulation of the pH and of the milieu within the body. They are a deciding factor in the absorption of vitamin B_{12}. Approximately 80% of the body's defence system is situated in the lymph follicles (*Peyer's patches*) of the GAT (gut associated tissue). These are just a few of the most important known functions. In the course of this section, I will point out others, especially the important psychological factor. Understandably intestinal therapy is a very intimate subject connected with many taboos. The consequences of intestinal therapy can often be far-reaching physically as well as psychologically. This presents a serious challenge for the therapist and for the patient. Both trust on the part of the patient and sensitivity on the part of the therapist are required.

It is a fact that a very large part of the population suffers from intestinal problems. I estimate that two-thirds have problems with their intestines, women more than men. Often these patients have not been able to find help for decades and therefore in the course of time accept the problem as inevitable.
The most frequent intestinal disorders are functional disorders such as irritable bowel syndrome (flatulence, stool irregularities, vague abdominal pains); inflammation of the intestines such as Crohn's disease or ulcerative colitis; or life-threatening diseases such as colorectal carcinoma. The most frequent diseases in practice are functional disorders. I will therefore concentrate here on these problems. The therapy of fungal disorders is very important in connection with this.

Many therapists use the term intestinal *sanitation* very carelessly. If we ask them more specifically we find that they treat more or less arbitrarily using a few single remedies. The symptoms often improve for a short time when treating in this way. But after a few weeks or after discontinuing the remedies the situation is the same as it was before treatment. I don't agree with this way of working. Sometimes this is done only to satisfy the patient momentarily or to avoid admitting that the therapist has no experience in treating this problem. Experience is invaluable when treating intestinal problems. You need many years to realise which problems are related to the intestines and which reactions are to be expected when you treat a patient with intestinal disorders, especially psychological reactions.

My viewpoint on this subject therefore corresponds to my general stand that not many treatments deserve the term intestinal *sanitation*. Intestinal *sanitation* is a far-reaching therapy which can perhaps stretch over years and involves as many areas of the body as possible. The aim of therapy is not only to remove supposedly harmful intestinal germs but in keeping with Enderlein's philosophy to fundamentally redevelop the whole milieu in the body. This enables the body to regulate its functions fully and properly again.

Procedure in Practice

Patients with intestinal disorders can suffer from very clear symptoms as well as from very vague symptoms. The greater the range of symptoms the more likely it is that the intestines are involved. Besides flatulence, a bloated feeling and constipation or diarrhoea as main symptoms there can be skin phenomena, hair problems, itching, migraines, frequent infections, urinary tract infections, vaginal mycosis and also sometimes fatigue, a decrease in energy, insomnia or further symptoms. Many patients have already undergone a coloscopy but this gives no insight to functional disorders and is rarely helpful in therapy.

If you have a darkfield microscope you can find clear clues to existing intestinal disorders sometimes even before the patient himself suffers from them.

The second measure to confirm the diagnosis is a stool examination carried out by a microbiological laboratory. A conventional stool examination is completely worthless as they only test for occult blood.

To improve the quality of the results when taking and sending a stool sample the patient should regard certain rules: The stool should not go into the toilet. Therefore it should be collected with paper or in a container. The fresh sample should be sent at the beginning of the week. To improve the diagnosis of intestinal fungi the patient should do the following: three days before taking the stool sample the patient should drink a glass of water with a tablespoon of cider vinegar spread over the day or eat a forkful of fresh sauerkraut before each meal. Both cause any bacteria present to detach themselves from the intestinal mucous membrane and thus help a correct diagnosis to be made. In addition an oral swab examination will improve the results of the stool examination by up to 50% because the oral mucosa is the first part of the digestive system.

A further measure is an examination of the patient's teeth and, depending on their condition, to refer the patient to a dentist who is aware of the biological situation in the body and who is good at his craft. Unfortunately it is very difficult to even find a dentist who halfway meets these requirements. Many dentists still consider amalgam as harmless let alone take into account the widely recognised fact that gum diseases are always related to intestinal problems. Intestinal therapy requires working closely together with a good dentist. Often I only begin intestinal therapy once the teeth have been seen to (amalgam removed, parodontosis treated, root problems treated, "dead teeth" i.e. root-treated teeth removed). The relationship between the teeth and certain organs in the body is already recognised. Accordingly, dental problems can cause pathogenic changes in the intestines, and intestinal problems can cause gum disease.

The next step is a urine test for toxic metals to find out the levels of toxic metals in the patient's body. This can be done by testing the urine using a suitable procedure. The importance of toxic metals in the body is based on research by the Swiss doctor Dr. Thomas Rau: fungi are known to be able to bind inorganic metals. As nothing in nature occurs without reason he assumes that fungi in the body can also bind inorganic metals and that they will try to solve any existing toxic metal problem for their host. They are therefore not the cause of the illness but a result of the problem. A therapy which aims to get rid of the fungi without taking into account the toxic metal poisoning therefore goes against nature and is doomed to fail. A further problem of toxic metals is that they cause therapy blockades which are impossible to break through no matter how good the biological remedies you use are.

All the examination results together form the basis for a promising intestinal therapy. In some cases an additional conventional medical examination may be necessary.

The remedies used

The SANUM remedies have proved over the years to be very effective for intestinal *sanitation*. Relapses are rare if the patient keeps to the guidelines as far as possible. I will therefore concentrate primarily on these remedies in my therapy plan. Only in long-standing cases do I sometimes use other remedies such as *Myrrhinil* from *Repha* or *Galivert, Heralvent* and *Oricant* from *Lühr-Lehrs* to maintain stimulation. In addition there is a whole range of plant based remedies which you can use.

The isopathic SANUM preparations for intestinal problems:

Remedies	Indication
UTILIN	for chronic inflammations and to activate specific defence system
RECARCIN	for chronic inflammations and to activate specific defence system
LATENSIN	for chronic inflammations (especially of the intestinal tract) and to activate specific defence system
NOTAKEHL	for inflammations and to enhance stimulation
FORTAKEHL	for the intestinal flora, for gastritis, enteritis, colitis, stomach ulcers, mycosis
SANKOMBI	for reversion of the *endobiont*
ALBICANSAN	for treatment of mycoses in general
PEFRAKEHL	for mycoses particularly caused by candida fungi
EXMYKEHL	for intestinal and vaginal fungal problems
NIGERSAN	for mould fungi (e.g. Aspergillus niger)

After many years of experience, my viewpoint is that colon hydro therapy is extremely advantageous in the treatment of intestinal problems. It is a well-known fact that the intestinal flora is very constant and well-established from birth onwards. Disturbances of the intestinal flora, a dysbiosis, are caused mainly by antibiotics, cortisone, oestrogen, antacids, food preservatives, toxic metals and laxative abuse. Especially pathogenic germs have an extraordinary ability to colonise and adhere to the intestinal mucosa. It is therefore an illusion to believe that you can decisively influence the intestinal situation by just taking a couple of remedies. Practice shows that patients treated this way have often taken intestinal *sanitation* remedies for years and nothing has happened.

Colon hydro therapy has proved to be very useful in such cases. A 45-minute irrigation combined with a specific massage of the lower abdomen relieves the intestines of old deposits. This upsets the well-established order within the intestines. The water masses cause chaos within the intestines and thus force the organism to find a new arrangement. This is necessary for a successful therapy. Colon hydro therapy regenerates the mucosa of the intestines, supports the redevelopment of the intestinal flora, enhances the body's defence system and produces more energy and a feeling of well-being in general. Colon hydro therapy is only contraindicated when treating acute or chronic inflammations such as Crohn's disease or ulcerative colitis. When treating patients suffering from heart diseases, care should be taken due to the loss of minerals.

Candida - a controversial topic

It is always claimed, especially by conventional medicine, that everybody has candida fungi in their body and that therefore treatment is not necessary. It is true that candida fungi are always in the body, but candida fungi are potentially pathogenic microbes which can cause illnesses. They can be responsible for a lot of disturbances. The body's defence system should therefore take suitable measures. When fungi are found in a stool examination this means that the body's defence system let them pass without killing them. We therefore have not only the problem of candida fungi but also the problem of a deficient immune system. In my experience the presence of candida fungi is confirmed in 50% of the patients who consult me. The necessity to treat candida is proved by the fact that the patients feel significantly better after therapy.

An extreme situation for me was a woman teacher (45) a few years ago. Her state of health was so bad that she seriously considered retiring early. The result of the stool examination showed a high level of candida fungi. After a few weeks of intensive therapy most of her symptoms had disappeared. She is now full of energy and one of my most thankful patients.

Basic information concerning candida fungi:
The yeast fungus *Candida albicans* occurs in two different forms (Dimorphism), as a single cell (yeast) and as mycelium (fungus) (⇨ *Cyclogenie!*):

Single cell (yeast) = facultative pathogenic,
is able to cause skin or mucosa lesions

In certain conditions, such as a weakened immune system or because of antibiotics, cortisone, or oestrogen the yeast cell can evolve and become increasingly pathogenic. The host cell dies. The yeast cell becomes a

Pseudo mycelium (fungus) = parasitic, invasive,
can cause lesions of tissues by penetration

Nystatin - yes or no?

The treatment of fungi problems in the intestines using the remedy *Nystatin* is still a controversial topic. I am horrified to still meet naturopaths who use *Nystatin* as a matter of course. In my opinion this is wrong. Prescribing *Nystatin* as an antimycotic is no better than using antibiotics against bacteria. It is often claimed that *Nystatin* is not absorbed by the body and is therefore not harmful in any way. I could accept this reasoning perhaps from a conventional doctor but in no way from a naturopath. It is just not the right way to solve the problem. *Nystatin* IS absorbed! The intestines of a patient suffering from intestinal disorders are not in a normal healthy condition. In this case the intestinal mucosa is inflamed and therefore permeable to bigger molecules including *Nystatin*. This is called *Leaky Gut Syndrome*. *Nystatin*, perhaps harmless in itself, is no longer harmless when it is able to penetrate into other body regions.

The assertion that using *Nystatin* does not cause any side effects is not correct either. *Nystatin* may kill a lot of the fungi present. These have to be eliminated by the body's immune system and the excretory organs. The patient will therefore inevitably suffer problems. A couple of weeks later the fungal problem will also be back since the root cause has not been dealt with. The opinion that solving the fungal problem by using *Nystatin* and a "diet against fungi" is logically an illusion. It just is not that simple. Therefore, neither am I in favour of the often praised diet against fungi.

The diet against fungi

Diet is an essential factor in the context of every therapy. Both the idea of killing the fungi by starving them of food and the idea of killing them with a couple of pills is an illusion. This just does not work. On the contrary. If I withdraw the food source from the fungi completely I force them to look around for other possibilities of nutrition. Thus, there is a risk that they will penetrate the intestinal mucosa membrane with the aid of proteolytic (protein digesting) enzymes. After this, the fungi enter the bloodstream and can cause mycotic disorders in different organs of the body. Therefore, it is contraindicated to fast when there is a candida infection!

Candida fungi only feed on sugar and prefer a putrefactive milieu, which is mainly caused by animal protein. The therapy therefore requires:

- no refined sugar or products with refined sugar
- no white flour or products with white flour
- reduction of animal protein in diet to a minimum
  i.e. less meat, eggs, dairy products

The plan for intestinal therapy

I created the following therapy plan for intestinal disorders over a number of years and tested it in practice. During this time I continually changed this plan. Eventually I was satisfied and have now been treating patients according to this plan for many years without any major changes. Only if the stool examination shows a rare disorder such as mould fungi (e.g. *Aspergillus niger*) may I adapt my plan slightly. This plan has proved incredibly reliable and successful in thousands of cases.

As you can see, I use a relatively large number of remedies in intestinal therapy. This is often not easy for the patient, particularly if he has only taken very little medication in his life up to this point. The therapy plan for taking the remedies is therefore clearly ordered. I hand it over to the patient combined with the prescription for the remedies. Thus, the patient can see at any time of the treatment exactly when and how he should use the remedies. It is often favourable for men, if their wives supervise this. Often the patients ask why so many remedies are necessary. I then explain that their intestinal flora has been disturbed for years or even decades. This unfavourable situation has become firmly established in their body. If I want to change this, I have to work on a relatively wide scale.

<u>My therapy is in keeping with SANUM therapy in general:</u>

1. Preparation of the milieu using **ALKALA N**
2. Stimulation and mucosal therapy using bacterial isopathic preparations **UTILIN**, **RECARCIN** and **LATENSIN**
3. Regulation therapy using **FORTAKEHL**, **PEFRAKEHL** and **SANKOMBI**
4. Redevelopment of the intestinal flora using the available remedies (⇨ plan)

If the candida diagnosis is negative I use the same therapy plan but without the remedy PEFRAKEHL. If the laboratory examination identifies mould fungi, such as *Aspergillus niger*, I additionally use the remedy NIGERSAN. *Spirulina*, which appears in my therapy plan, is produced from algae. It is well known that algae like fungi are able to bind inorganic toxic metals and thus enable the body to excrete these. Besides, *Spirulina* contains approx. 60% vegetable protein which is biologically available for the body, and in addition it contains valuable organic minerals and numerous vitamins. This advantageously supports the therapy as a whole.

Mutaflor is in my view an important remedy in connection with intestinal therapy. A short explanation: the German doctor *Dr. Alfred Nissle* observed during World War I that all soldiers in his company apart from one had fallen ill with dysentery. He examined the intestinal flora of this soldier and found a divergent coli bacterium which obviously prevented this soldier from falling ill. He isolated this germ and from it developed the remedy *Mutaflor*. *Mutaflor* today still contains the same live coli bacterium which *Dr. Nissle* discovered in 1917. It speaks for the quality of this bacterium that it has not changed or developed pathogenic qualities in the course of more than 80 years.

The isopathic remedy SANUVIS included in the plan, contains potentised L(+) lactic acid and is used to improve the situation in the small intestines. Eating yoghurt is by comparison not very effective therapeutically. Eating a forkful of raw sauerkraut before each meal is far more effective. Related to this topic, I do not believe in constantly introducing large quantities of foreign strains of bacteria or fungi into the body, such as are in kombucha or kefir.

Of course there are also other possibilities for an intestinal therapy. Personally I only treat according to the given plan. Thus, today I am no longer prepared to only do half or three-quarters of an intestinal treatment. I am not willing to make compromises. We have been treating patients very successfully according to this therapy for more than 10 years. An intestinal *sanitation* is not a therapy of 4 or 6 weeks either. Sometimes this is possible. On the other hand it can last for 1 or 2 years. This is asking a lot of the patient. He needs to be patient. Initial exacerbation is far more frequent within the first weeks than instant improvements, but this is considered to be a healing reaction.

The plan for intestinal *sanitation* with candida fungi present

date		morning	lunchtime	evening	directions
	1st day	**LATENSIN 4X** 1 capsule			**LATENSIN, RECARCIN, UTILIN** on an empty stomach in the morning, open capsule and spread contents under the tongue, after this eat and drink nothing for 1 hour
		ALKALA N acc. to directions	**ALKALA N** acc. to directions	**ALKALA N** acc. to directions	**ALKALA N** drink a glass of water with a level measuring spoon of **ALKALA N**, 1/3 of this glass before each meal. Drink this glass of **ALKALA N** despite the fact that the indicator sticks in the pack show a blue colour from the 2nd day onwards.
		Spirulina 3 tablets with meal	**Spirulina** 3 tablets with meal	**Spirulina** 3 tablets with meal	**Spirulina** should be taken every day until the jar is empty. Then a new test for toxic metals is necessary.
	2nd day	**ALKALA N** acc. to directions	**ALKALA N** acc. to directions	**ALKALA N** acc. to directions	
	3rd day	**UTILIN 4X** 1 capsule **ALKALA N** acc. to directions	**ALKALA N** acc. to directions	**ALKALA N** acc. to directions	
	4th day	**ALKALA N** acc. to directions	**ALKALA N** acc. to directions	**ALKALA N** acc. to directions	
	5th day	**RECARCIN 4X** 1 capsule **ALKALA N** acc. to directions	**ALKALA N** acc. to directions	**ALKALA N** acc. to directions	
	6th day	**ALKALA N** acc. to directions	**ALKALA N** acc. to directions	**ALKALA N** acc. to directions	
	7th day	**LATENSIN 4X** 1 capsule **ALKALA N** acc. to directions	**ALKALA N** acc. to directions	**ALKALA N** acc. to directions	
	8th day	**ALKALA N** acc. to directions	**ALKALA N** acc. to directions	**ALKALA N** acc. to directions	
	9th day	**UTILIN 4X** 1 capsule **ALKALA N** acc. to directions	**ALKALA N** acc. to directions	**ALKALA N** acc. to directions	
	10th day	**ALKALA N** acc. to directions	**ALKALA N** acc. to directions	**ALKALA N** acc. to directions	

date		morning	lunchtime	evening	directions
	11th day	**RECARCIN 4X** 1 capsule **ALKALA N** acc. to directions	**ALKALA N** acc. to directions	**ALKALA N** acc. to directions	
	12th day	**ALKALA N** acc. to directions	**ALKALA N** acc. to directions	**ALKALA N** acc. to directions	
	13th day	**LATENSIN 4X** 1 capsule **ALKALA N** acc. to directions	**ALKALA N** acc. to directions	**ALKALA N** acc. to directions	
	14th day	**ALKALA N** acc. to directions	**ALKALA N** acc. to directions	**ALKALA N** acc. to directions	
	15th day	**FORTAKEHL 5X** 8 drops acc. to directions **UTILIN 4X** 1 capsule **Mutaflor 20 mg** 1 capsule with meal **SANUVIS** 1 tablet with meal	**SANKOMBI 5X** 8 drops acc. to directions **SANUVIS** 1 tablet with meal	**PEFRAKEHL 5X** 8 drops acc. to directions **Mutaflor 20 mg** 1 capsule with meal **SANUVIS** 1 tablet with meal	**FORTAKEHL** on an empty stomach in the morning, 8 drops before breakfast put on dry bread and chew until it is fluid, after this eat and drink nothing for 1 hour: When you take a capsule on the same day take this immediately afterwards and do not eat or drink anything for 1 hour **SANKOMBI, PEFRAKEHL** 4 drops draw from the back of the hand into each nostril,
	16th day	**FORTAKEHL 5X** 8 drops acc. to directions **Mutaflor 20 mg** **SANUVIS**	**SANKOMBI 5X** 8 drops acc. to directions **SANUVIS** 1 tablet with meal	**PEFRAKEHL 5X** 8 drops acc. to directions **Mutaflor 20 mg** **SANUVIS**	
	17th day	**FORTAKEHL 5X** 8 drops acc. to directions **RECARCIN 4X** 1 capsule **Mutaflor 20 mg** **SANUVIS**	**SANKOMBI 5X** 8 drops acc. to directions **SANUVIS** 1 tablet with meal	**PEFRAKEHL 5X** 8 drops acc. to directions **Mutaflor 20 mg** **SANUVIS**	
	18th day	**FORTAKEHL 5X** 8 drops acc. to directions **Mutaflor 20 mg** **SANUVIS**	**SANKOMBI 5X** 8 drops acc. to directions **SANUVIS** 1 tablet with meal	**PEFRAKEHL 5X** 8 drops acc. to directions **Mutaflor 20 mg** **SANUVIS**	
	19th day	**FORTAKEHL 5X** 8 drops acc. to directions **LATENSIN 4X** 1 capsule **Mutaflor 20 mg** **SANUVIS**	**SANKOMBI 5X** 8 drops acc. to directions **SANUVIS** 1 tablet with meal	**PEFRAKEHL 5X** 8 drops acc. to directions **Mutaflor 20 mg** **SANUVIS**	
	20th day	**FORTAKEHL 5X** 8 drops acc. to directions **Mutaflor 20 mg** **SANUVIS**	**SANKOMBI 5X** 8 drops acc. to directions **SANUVIS** 1 tablet with meal	**PEFRAKEHL 5X** 8 drops acc. to directions **Mutaflor 20 mg** **SANUVIS**	
	21st day	**FORTAKEHL 5X** 8 drops acc. to directions **UTILIN 4X** 1 capsule **Mutaflor 20 mg** **SANUVIS**	**SANKOMBI 5X** 8 drops acc. to directions **SANUVIS** 1 tablet with meal	**PEFRAKEHL 5X** 8 drops acc. to directions **Mutaflor 20 mg** **SANUVIS**	
	22nd day	**FORTAKEHL 5X** 8 drops acc. to directions **Mutaflor 20 mg** **SANUVIS**	**SANKOMBI 5X** 8 drops acc. to directions **SANUVIS** 1 tablet with meal	**PEFRAKEHL 5X** 8 drops acc. to directions **Mutaflor 20 mg** **SANUVIS**	

date		morning	lunchtime	evening	directions
	23rd day	**FORTAKEHL 5X** 8 drops acc. to directions **RECARCIN 4X** 1 capsule **Mutaflor 20 mg** **SANUVIS**	**SANKOMBI 5X** 8 drops acc. to directions **SANUVIS** 1 tablet with meal	**PEFRAKEHL 5X** 8 drops acc. to directions **Mutaflor 20 mg** **SANUVIS**	
	24th day	**FORTAKEHL 5X** 8 drops acc. to directions **Mutaflor 20 mg** **SANUVIS**	**SANKOMBI 5X** 8 drops acc. to directions **SANUVIS** 1 tablet with meal	**PEFRAKEHL 5X** 8 drops acc. to directions **Mutaflor 20 mg** **SANUVIS**	
	25th day	**FORTAKEHL 5X** 8 drops acc. to directions **LATENSIN 4X** 1 capsule **Mutaflor 100 mg** **SANUVIS**	**SANKOMBI 5X** 8 drops acc. to directions **SANUVIS** 1 tablet with meal	**PEFRAKEHL 5X** 8 drops acc. to directions **Mutaflor 100 mg** **SANUVIS**	
	26th day	**FORTAKEHL 5X** 8 drops acc. to directions **Mutaflor 100 mg** **SANUVIS**	**SANKOMBI 5X** 8 drops acc. to directions **SANUVIS** 1 tablet with meal	**PEFRAKEHL 5X** 8 drops acc. to directions **Mutaflor 100 mg** **SANUVIS**	
	27th day	**FORTAKEHL 5X** 8 drops acc. to directions **UTILIN 4X** 1 Capsule **Mutaflor 100 mg** **SANUVIS**	**SANKOMBI 5X** 8 drops acc. to directions **SANUVIS** 1 tablet with meal	**PEFRAKEHL 5X** 8 drops acc. to directions **Mutaflor 100 mg** **SANUVIS**	
	28th day	**FORTAKEHL 5X** 8 drops acc. to directions **Mutaflor 100 mg** **SANUVIS**	**SANKOMBI 5X** 8 drops acc. to directions **SANUVIS** 1 tablet with meal	**PEFRAKEHL 5X** 8 drops acc. to directions **Mutaflor 100 mg** **SANUVIS**	
	29th day	**FORTAKEHL 5X** 8 drops acc. to directions **RECARCIN 4X** 1 capsule **Mutaflor 100 mg** **SANUVIS**	**SANKOMBI 5X** 8 drops acc. to directions **SANUVIS** 1 tablet with meal	**PEFRAKEHL 5X** 8 drops acc. to directions **Mutaflor 100 mg** **SANUVIS**	
	30th day	**FORTAKEHL 5X** 8 drops acc. to directions **Mutaflor 100 mg** **SANUVIS**	**SANKOMBI 5X** 8 drops acc. to directions **SANUVIS** 1 tablet with meal	**PEFRAKEHL 5X** 8 drops acc. to directions **Mutaflor 100 mg** **SANUVIS**	
	31st day	**FORTAKEHL 5X** 8 drops acc. to directions **Mutaflor 100 mg** **SANUVIS**	**SANKOMBI 5X** 8 drops acc. to directions **SANUVIS** 1 tablet with meal	**PEFRAKEHL 5X** 8 drops acc. to directions **Mutaflor 100 mg** **SANUVIS**	
	32nd day	**FORTAKEHL 5X** 8 drops acc. to directions **Mutaflor 100 mg** **SANUVIS**	**SANKOMBI 5X** 8 drops acc. to directions **SANUVIS** 1 tablet with meal	**PEFRAKEHL 5X** 8 drops acc. to directions **Mutaflor 100 mg** **SANUVIS**	
	33rd day	**FORTAKEHL 5X** 8 drops acc. to directions **Mutaflor 100 mg** **SANUVIS**	**SANKOMBI 5X** 8 drops acc. to directions **SANUVIS** 1 tablet with meal	**PEFRAKEHL 5X** 8 drops acc. to directions **Mutaflor 100 mg** **SANUVIS**	
	34th day	**FORTAKEHL 5X** 8 drops acc. to directions **Mutaflor 100 mg** **SANUVIS**	**SANKOMBI 5X** 8 drops acc. to directions **SANUVIS** 1 tablet with meal	**PEFRAKEHL 5X** 8 drops acc. to directions **Mutaflor 100 mg** **SANUVIS**	**FORTAKEHL, SANKOMBI, PEFRAKEHL, SANUVIS** Take until bottle or pack is empty
all remedies - besides ALKALA N - take until pack or bottle is empty					

Therapy of stomach problems

A lot of patients, mainly men, come primarily because of stomach problems, not because of intestinal problems. In this case it is still helpful, after a conventional medical check-up if necessary, to begin therapy by first treating the intestines. Experience has shown that the stomach problems often disappear as soon as the intestines have been sorted out.

In connection with this, I want to mention two further topics: helicobacter pylori and antacids. Nowadays helicobacter pylori is considered responsible for all problems related to the stomach, including gastric cancer. It should not be necessary to write any more on this topic. Once again we have found a scapegoat but I believe that helicobacter pylori is only the result of the problem and not the cause. Anybody who halfway understands Enderlein's philosophy must be able to realise this. On the other hand, helicobacter pylori enables conventional medicine to do what they always do: to use antibiotics. Before starting therapy with antibiotics it is necessary to use antacids to reduce gastric acid. This measure is a disadvantage for the patient because the gastric cells which produce gastric acid at the same time produce four or five times the amount of the alkaline buffer substance $NaHCO_3$. By buffering gastric acid using antacids alkaline deficiencies inevitably arise. Antacids are the most widely bought prescription-free medication on the market! You only have to read the long list of possible side effects to question the wisdom of this. They can affect eyesight, hearing, every possible organ and organ system in the body and even lead to anaphylaxis. As said: prescription-free!

Checking of the therapy results

Three months after an intestinal treatment you should check the blood under a dark-field microscope, organise a stool examination and test the urine for toxic metals. Depending on the results, therapy is finished or it should be repeated or adapted. You will have a lot of success using this therapy concept. If in rare cases you are not successful despite all your efforts and the best therapy look for undiscovered therapy blockades such as conventional medication which the patient is taking. Or try to find out why the patient "needs" his intestinal problem.

The intestines and their psychological importance

The whole digestive system is, as is well known, very closely related to the way we try to solve our mental and emotional problems. It is important to go into this a little deeper as you will often be confronted with this problem in practice.

Patients with gastric problems are mostly male. They are critical, often over-critical, of others and themselves and dependent on the opinion of other people. These patients always try to achieve a maximum of success in order to receive the necessary recognition.

Patients with intestinal problems are generally female. They tend to suppress their problems, this means to "swallow" them. Men are often able to let off steam by doing sports, watching football on television or going down to the pub. Women today are still forced to play the role of a loving wife and mother for their family to the point of collapse.

Thus, the intestines receive not only garbage from the wrong diet but as a result of permanent frustration "*emotional garbage*", too. You can be sure that this burden will come to the fore during therapy and then present a great challenge for both the therapist and the patient. The patients thus have the chance to look at their problems once again. If it is possible, they should not try to suppress their problems again. The decision whether the intestinal problems can be permanently changed for the better is often made at this point.

Horvi Therapy

The *Horvi* remedies include the enzymes of the poison of snakes, toads, spiders and other similar animals. In my opinion *Horvi* is the ideal therapy in specific cases such as cysts or myoma of the womb or sometimes in cases which do not respond to other therapies. Operations are often no longer necessary after *Horvi* therapy. Working with *Horvi* remedies is not straightforward so I always request a therapy plan from the *Horvi* company before I start treatment. *Horvi* therapy can cause certain side effects. Local pains in the injection area or itching over the whole body appear very frequently but only temporarily.

Horvi remedies are available as ampoules or drops.

> Practice case: female patient, 54
>
> The patient has had a large lipoma on her shoulder for many years
> (size: 11 x 14 cm and 4-5 cm high).
>
> According to the individual therapy plan from *Horvi* I infiltrated the remedies with a small needle into several spots around the edge of the lipoma (not into the lipoma itself). Within two months the lipoma had decreased in size by about a third. We will continue treatment until the lipoma has disappeared completely.

Large lipoma are often inoperable and *Horvi* therapy is therefore the only alternative for these patients.

The unpopular subject of diet

Diet was of utmost importance to Enderlein. Many therapists unfortunately do not like hearing this. I have already mentioned that Enderlein was not only a strict vegetarian but also mainly ate raw vegetables! That does not necessarily mean that everybody has to live on a frugal diet of raw vegetables. Most of us believe though that we can eat whatever we like, smoke and drink as much as we like and still stay healthy. That this is not possible is evident.

Nobody would dream of giving his beloved car diesel when it needs petrol, but this is exactly what we do with our bodies every day. I do not advocate a particular dietary philosophy. It must be obvious that one single diet cannot be suitable for everybody. We are individuals with completely individual dispositions and needs. No two people are the same. A person who works on a building site has different needs compared to a person who works at a computer in an office. Further factors to be considered are the person's social needs and what they do in their free time. Only a diet that takes all this into account is the right one for that particular person.

Diet has always been the most important factor for the milieu. There is no way around this. This means that we have to find, together with the patient, a diet that meets the individual needs of this person. This is possible but the patient usually has great difficulties in putting it into practice. Often the whole social environment is hostile to change.

I think it is generally wrong to consume a lot of processed foods and instant products, but unfortunately many people nowadays do exactly this. The food industry has absolutely no scruples and confronts us with a great number of chemical additives, all of which at some time damage the organism in some form. (⇨ Literature: H.-U. Grimm, "Die Suppe lügt")

Blood Group Diet
according to Dr. Peter J. D'Adamo

A rather useful clue to a suitable diet is provided in my opinion by the research of the American doctor Dr. D'Adamo. According to him the blood group is the basic characteristic that has hardly changed over millennia! Our body is therefore poorly adapted to the demands of modern life! This is why we have such problems with numerous germs. But these are not the problem - we ourselves are the problem!

According to Dr. D'Adamo, and my own experience corroborates this, people with blood group 0 often have difficulties with dairy products, particularly milk. People with blood group A often have problems with meat and also with dairy products (they are natural vegetarians!). The only blood group that can properly digest milk and other dairy products is B (mainly eastern Europeans and Asians).

As this aspect is very important to me, I have worked for many years with the AB0 test sera from *Johnson & Johnson* and have a result within 5 minutes. This means the patient can start with dietary changes immediately.

Water - our most important nutrient

Water is doubtlessly our most important requirement. We know that we need daily approx. 2 l of water depending on our age, size, weight and diet. No other nutrient is consumed in this quantity. Opinions on what kind of water we should use differ. It is constantly being claimed that our tap water is the most tested nutrient. At the beginning of each therapy I test the patient's urine and the tap or mineral water they consume for toxic metals. When testing we find that tap water is as a rule contaminated with inorganic toxic metals such as copper, zinc or mercury. (Often chlorine, fluorine and other toxic substances have been added too.) These inorganic metals are toxic. They also block biological therapies such as SANUM therapy. The WHO (*World Health Organisation*) claims that a high percentage of today's illnesses are caused by toxic-metals. I therefore think that it is absolutely necessary to make this situation clear and to take suitable measures.

Many patients use boiled tap water for coffee and tea. Boiling may kill any bacteria present but logically does not eliminate toxic metals. In Germany we often drink carbonated mineral water. It usually contains a lot of inorganic minerals which the body can rarely use. They must therefore be excreted. If this is not possible the body deposits them somewhere in the body, which is not beneficial to our health.

A special topic in Germany are the so-called bottled "healing waters". Thus a particularly well-known spa ("healing") water contains:

602.5 mg	sodium
122.0 mg	calcium
28.1 mg	potassium
1472 mg	carbonic acid

I would consider it irresponsible to let a patient who is suffering from heart-circulatory disorders drink such a mineral water. In my opinion this is not a healing water, this is a salt solution! French spring water often contains less than 20 mg minerals in total.

Carbonic acid is an excretion product of the human body. For example, we excrete volatile acids from fruits via the respiratory tract. I do not think it is wise to consume something which is basically an excretion product. Strangely enough you will find non-carbonated oligo-mineral water, which contains minimal amounts of minerals, in most other countries in the world. It is only the Germans who are still on the "mineral water trip" i.e. they still believe in the goodness of carbonated mineral water. Again and again, I am shocked, that it is often not possible in so-called "good" restaurants to be served a spring water with low mineral contents and without carbonic acid. This is a matter of course in France or Italy.

Ultimately we are then confronted with the question: where do I find a water of optimal quality? After more than ten years of researching this subject I have come to the conclusion that reverse osmosis is the most practical solution. This process filters out all toxic substances, bacteria and viruses with a 100% reliability. The built-in membrane does not absorb the undesired substances unlike the widely used active-charcoal filters. It is continually rinsed clean so that it is always 100% effective. The appliance also revitalises the water according to Dr. Aschoff. Appliances for household use are not exorbitant and I therefore recommend them to my patients.

References

Dr. med. Maria-M. Bleker "Blood Examination in Darkfield"

Dr. med. Niels Krack "Die Nasale Reflex-Therapie"

Dr. Peter J. D'Adamo / Catherine Whitney "Live Right 4 Your Type"

Literature

"Blood Examination in Darkfield" (German and English)
Dr. med. Maria-M. Bleker
Semmelweis-Verlag ISBN 3-925524-01-0

"Introduction into darkfield diagnostics" (English)
Dr. Cornelia Schwerdtle & Franz Arnoul
Semmelweis-Verlag

"Die Nasale Reflex-Therapie" (German)
Dr. med. Niels Krack
Haug-Verlag ISBN 3-830-40680-0

"Live Right 4 Your Type" (English)
Peter J. D'Adamo, Catherine Whitney
Michael Joseph ISBN: 0399146733

"Die Suppe lügt" (German)
Hans-Ulrich Grimm
Klett-Cotta ISBN 3-608-93685-8